Anal Canal Cancers

Editor

CATHY ENG

SURGICAL ONCOLOGY CLINICS OF NORTH AMERICA

www.surgonc.theclinics.com

Consulting Editor
NICHOLAS J. PETRELLI

January 2017 • Volume 26 • Number 1

ELSEVIER

1600 John F. Kennedy Boulevard • Suite 1800 • Philadelphia, Pennsylvania, 19103-2899

http://www.theclinics.com

SURGICAL ONCOLOGY CLINICS OF NORTH AMERICA Volume 26, Number 1
January 2017 ISSN 1055-3207, ISBN-13: 978-0-323-48272-1

Editor: John Vassallo (j.vassallo@elsevier.com)
Developmental Editor: Meredith Clinton

Surgical Oncology Clinics of North America (ISSN 1055-3207) is published quarterly by Elsevier Inc., 360 Park Avenue South, New York, NY 10010-1710. Months of publication are January, April, July, and October. Business and Editorial Offices: 1600 John F. Kennedy Blvd., Ste. 1800, Philadelphia, PA 19103-2899. Customer Service Office: 3251 Riverport Lane, Maryland Heights, MO 63043. Periodicals postage paid at New York, NY and additional mailing offices. Subscription prices are $296.00 per year (US individuals), $490.00 (US institutions) $100.00 (US student/resident), $337.00 (Canadian individuals), $620.00 (Canadian institutions), $205.00 (Canadian student/resident), $418.00 (foreign individuals), $620.00 (foreign institutions), and $205.00 (foreign student/resident). Foreign air speed delivery is included in all *Clinics* subscription prices. All prices are subject to change without notice. **POSTMASTER**: Send address changes to *Surgical Oncology Clinics of North America*, Elsevier Health Science Division, Subscription Customer Service, 3251 Riverport Lane, Maryland Heights, MO 63043. **Customer Service: 1-800-654-2452 (US and Canada). 314-447-8871 (outside US and Canada). Fax: 314-447-8029. E-mail: journalscustomerservice-usa@elsevier.com (for print support); journalsonline support-usa@elsevier.com (for online support).**

Reprints. For copies of 100 or more, of articles in this publication, please contact the Commercial Reprints Department, Elsevier Inc., 360 Park Avenue South, New York, New York 10010-1710. Tel. 212-633-3874; Fax: 212-633-3820; E-mail: reprints@elsevier.com.

Surgical Oncology Clinics of North America is covered in *MEDLINE/PubMed (Index Medicus) and EMBASE/ Excerpta Medica, Current Contents/Clinical Medicine, and ISI/BIOMED.*

Contributors

CONSULTING EDITOR

NICHOLAS J. PETRELLI, MD, FACS
Bank of America Endowed Medical Director, Helen F. Graham Cancer Center & Research Institute, Christiana Care Health Systems, Newark, Delaware; Professor of Surgery, Thomas Jefferson University, Philadelphia, Pennsylvania

EDITOR

CATHY ENG, MD, FACP
Professor, Sophie Caroline Steves Distinguished Professor in Cancer Research, Associate Medical Director, Colorectal Center, The University of Texas MD Anderson Cancer Center, Department of Gastrointestinal Medical Oncology, Houston, Texas

AUTHORS

RICHARD ADAMS, BSc, BM BS, MRCP, FRCR, MD
Reader, Honorary Consultant in Clinical Oncology, Velindre Cancer Centre, Cardiff University, Cardiff, United Kingdom

DAVID ASTILL, BSc Hons, BMBS, PhD, FRCPA
Department of Anatomical Pathology, Flinders Medical Centre, Flinders University, Bedford Park, South Australia, Australia

AL B. BENSON III, MD
Hematology/Oncology, Department of Medicine, Robert H. Lurie Comprehensive Cancer Center, Feinberg School of Medicine, Northwestern University, Chicago, Illinois

GINA BROWN, MBBS, MRCP, FRCR
Professor of Gastrointestinal Cancer Imaging, Department of Radiology, The Royal Marsden Hospital, Imperial College, Sutton, United Kingdom

KRISTEN K. CIOMBOR, MD, MSCI
Assistant Professor, Department of Internal Medicine, Division of Medical Oncology, The Ohio State University, Columbus, Ohio

RENATA COUDRY, MD, PhD
Chief, Anatomic Pathology Department, Director of Molecular Pathology Laboratory, Hospital Sírio Libânes, São Paulo, São Paulo, Brasil

BRIAN G. CZITO, MD
Gary Hock and Lynn Proctor, Department of Radiation Oncology, Duke University Medical Center, Durham, North Carolina

CATHY ENG, MD, FACP
Professor, Sophie Caroline Steves Distinguished Professor in Cancer Research, Associate Medical Director, Colorectal Center, The University of Texas MD Anderson Cancer Center, Department of Gastrointestinal Medical Oncology, Houston, Texas

RANDY D. ERNST, MD
Professor, Department of Diagnostic Radiology, Division of Diagnostic Imaging, The University of Texas MD Anderson Cancer Center, Houston, Texas

ROB GLYNNE-JONES, FRCR, FRCP
Consultant Clinical Oncologist, Radiotherapy Department, Mount Vernon Centre for Cancer Treatment, Middlesex, United Kingdom

KIRSTEN GORMLY, MBBS, FRANZCR
Dr Jones & Partners Medical Imaging, Kurralta Park, South Australia, Australia

PAULO M. HOFF, MD, PhD, FACP
Professor of Oncology, Instituto do Câncer do Estado de São Paulo, Faculdade de Medicina da Universidade de São Paulo, São Paulo, São Paulo, Brasil

LISA A. KACHNIC, MD
Professor and Chair, Department of Radiation Oncology, Vanderbilt University Medical Center, Nashville, Tennessee

MICHELE LONGABAUGH, RN
Sr. Field Clinical Support, BIOTRONIK Inc., Lake Oswego, Oregon

ETHAN B. LUDMIR, MD
Resident, Department of Radiation Oncology, The University of Texas MD Anderson Cancer Center, Houston, Texas

CRAIG A. MESSICK, MD
Assistant Professor of Surgery, Section of Colon and Rectal Surgery, Surgical Oncology, The University of Texas MD Anderson Cancer Center, Houston, Texas

CAMILA MOTTA VENCHIARUTTI MONIZ, MD
Instituto do Câncer do Estado de São Paulo, Faculdade de Medicina da Universidade de São Paulo, São Paulo, São Paulo, Brasil

VAN MORRIS, MD
Assistant Professor, Department of Gastrointestinal Medical Oncology, The University of Texas MD Anderson Cancer Center, Houston, Texas

VALERIE M. NELSON, MD, MBA
Hematology/Oncology, Department of Medicine, Robert H. Lurie Comprehensive Cancer Center, Feinberg School of Medicine, Northwestern University, Chicago, Illinois

JOEL M. PALEFSKY, MD
Professor, Division of Infectious Diseases, Department of Medicine, University of California at San Francisco, San Francisco, California

SUSAN PENDLEBURY, MBBS, FRANZCR
Associate Professor, Genesis Health Care, St Vincent's Hospital, Sydney, New South Wales, Australia

SHEELA RAO, MD, FRCP
Consultant Medical Oncologist, Royal Marsden Hospital, London & Surrey, United Kingdom

MIGUEL A. RODRIGUEZ-BIGAS, MD, FACS, FASCRS
Section of Colon and Rectal Surgery, Professor, Division of Surgery, Department of
Surgical Oncology, The University of Texas MD Anderson Cancer Center, Houston, Texas

AMITESH C. ROY, MD, MSc, FRACP
Lecturer, Department of Medical Oncology, Flinders Centre For Innovation in Cancer,
Flinders Medical Centre, Flinders University, Bedford Park, South Australia, Australia

TARIK SAMMOUR, MBChB, FRACS, PhD
Colorectal Surgical Oncology Fellow, Division of Surgery, Department of Surgical
Oncology, The University of Texas MD Anderson Cancer Center, Houston, Texas

EVA SEGELOV, MBBS, PhD, FRACP
Associate Professor, St Vincent's Clinical School, St Vincent's Hospital, University of New
South Wales, Sydney, New South Wales, Australia

SIMRON SINGH, BSc, MD, MPH, FRCPC
Division of Medical Oncology, Odette Cancer Centre, Sunnybrook Health
Sciences Centre, Department of Medicine, University of Toronto, Toronto, Ontario,
Canada

JOHN M. SKIBBER, MD, FACS
Professor, Division of Surgery, Department of Surgical Oncology, The University of Texas
MD Anderson Cancer Center, Houston, Texas

JOSEPH SPARANO, MD
Professor of Medicine & Women's Health, Department of Oncology, Montefiore Medical
Center, Albert Einstein College of Medicine, Bronx, New York

CHIA-CHING J. WANG, MD
Clinical Instructor, Division of Hematology/Oncology, Department of Medicine,
Zuckerberg San Francisco General Hospital, San Francisco, California

DAVID WATTCHOW, BM BS, PhD, FRACS
Professor, Department of Surgery, Flinders Medical Centre, Flinders University, Bedford
Park, South Australia, Australia

Contents

I was diagnosed with rare anal cancer. As overwhelming as the diagnosis was, it was complicated by limited treatment infrastructure and clinical research, side-effect management, and lack of awareness and support organizations. Anal cancer encompasses so much more than receiving prescribed treatment and focusing on recovery. It requires patients to become experts on their disease, its treatment, and side effects. Even more challenging is finding support and advocacy. My experience has been difficult, complex, and arduous. It is hoped that this article will provide a voice for the many that have been silenced by stigma of anal cancer.

Anal cancer is a rare malignancy, although its incidence has been increasing in recent decades. This article discusses risk factors for anal cancer and how these risk factors affect the changing demographics of this disease.

Anal cancer is an increasingly common non–AIDS-defining cancer among individuals infected with the human immunodeficiency virus (HIV). It is associated with human papillomavirus (HPV). HPV16 is the most common genotype detected in anal cancers. The HPV types detected in anal cancer are included in the 9-valent vaccine. HPV vaccines have demonstrated efficacy in reducing anal precancerous lesions in HIV-infected individuals. Standard treatment has been fluorouracil and mitomycin (or cisplatin) plus radiation. Continued studies are needed to test new treatment strategies in HIV-infected patients with anal cancer to determine which treatment protocols provide the best therapeutic index.

Anal dysplasia is a cytopathology term describing specific squamous cell morphology and represents a varying degree of benign changes. Often a

Over the past several decades, clinical trials have demonstrated improved disease-related outcomes in the definitive treatment of anal cancer. Although treatment with radiation and concurrent chemotherapy results in high rates of cure, significant acute and late toxicities are seen. This review focuses on the evolution of treatment-related toxicity for anal cancer. Management of these adverse effects is reviewed, as are future directions in anal cancer treatment and their impact on toxicity.

Surgery for anal cancer is usually reserved for patients with persistent disease or local recurrence after definitive chemoradiation therapy. Patients with local recurrence should be re-evaluated for evidence of metastatic disease using positron emission tomography–computed tomography, and the local anatomy should be delineated with MRI. Eligible patients should undergo tailored surgery with the aim of achieving an R0 resection. Management is best undertaken within a specialized multidisciplinary setting. Careful patient selection and shared decision making are paramount for achieving acceptable patient-centered outcomes.

Anal squamous cell cancer is most frequently a locoregional disease that is amenable to curative therapy in a majority of fit patients. Complete response rates after chemoradiotherapy (CRT) are good, with up to 75% of patients with no evidence of relapse on surveillance. Relapse is most frequently locoregional and is often amenable to salvage surgery with curative intent. Effective surveillance attempts to improve outcomes by identifying recurrent or persistent disease early, managing both acute and late toxicities, and offering reassurance to patients. This article explores the rationale and evidence for surveillance programs after definitive CRT.

Squamous cell carcinoma of the anal canal (SCCA) represents an orphan disease. Although prior infection with human papilloma virus is associated with the development of SCCA, knowledge of this relationship has proven ineffective in identifying therapeutic agents that have activity in the management of metastatic SCCA. Combination chemotherapy with traditional cytotoxic agents has demonstrated efficacy in multiple small series. However, immune checkpoint blockade agents have demonstrated efficacy for patients with refractory metastatic SCCA; these agents hold promise in the horizon for patients with metastatic SCCA. Clinical trials should be considered for oncologists to manage patients with metastatic SCCA.

Uncommon neoplasms of the anal canal are associated with significant diagnostic dilemma in clinical practice and a high index of suspicion and pathologic expertise is needed. The incidence is likely to increase, particularly of small, incidental lesions found because of use of more frequent colonoscopy and high-definition MRI. Generally treatment follows that of the same histologic subtype in other anatomic location. Surgical intervention is the cornerstone for cure in early/localized disease; however, removal of the anal canal is associated with significant morbidities and quality of life issues. A centralized global registry/database established under the auspices of the International Rare Care Initiative collaboration would be useful.

SURGICAL ONCOLOGY
CLINICS OF NORTH AMERICA

RELATED INTEREST

Surgical Clinics of North America, December 2015 (Vol. 95, Issue 6)
Inflammatory Bowel Disease
Kerry L. Hammond, *Editor*
http://www.surgical.theclinics.com/

THE CLINICS ARE AVAILABLE ONLINE!
Access your subscription at:
www.theclinics.com

Foreword

Anal Cancer 2016

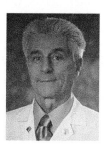

Nicholas J. Petrelli, MD, FACS
Consulting Editor

This issue of the *Surgical Oncology Clinics of North America* tackles the issue of carcinoma of the anal canal. The guest editor is Cathy Eng, MD, FACP. Dr Eng is the Sophie Caroline Steves Distinguished Professor in Cancer Research and Associate Medical Director of the Colorectal Center at the University of Texas MD Anderson Cancer Center. As stated in her preface, Dr Eng has gathered a multidisciplinary group of international renowned experts to provide their expertise on various topics of interest in cancer of the anal canal.

One example is an article entitled, "Epidemiology of Anal Canal Cancer," by Drs Nelson and Benson. Dr Al Benson from the Department of Medicine at the Robert H. Lurie Comprehensive Cancer Center at Northwestern University has a distinguished career in the treatment of gastrointestinal tumors and has been a major player in the National Cancer Institute clinical trials program. This article describes the incidence of anal canal cancer, which is increasing, and also the risk factors for this cancer. Another example is the article entitled, "Anal Dysplasia," by Drs Messick and Rodriguez-Bigas. Dr Rodriguez-Bigas is a talented surgical oncologist at the MD Anderson Cancer Center with expertise in anal, colon, and rectal cancer. Along with Drs Skibber and Sammour, Dr Rodriguez-Bigas is also a coauthor on an article entitled, "Locally Recurrent Disease Related to Anal Canal Cancers."

Along with the authors above, the 12 articles in this issue of the *Surgical Oncology Clinics of North America* extensively describe the gamut of anal canal carcinoma. With the increasing incidence in anal carcinoma, the timing of this issue of the *Surgical Oncology Clinics of North America* is perfect. It behooves practicing physicians and residents in training to utilize this issue as a reference for the treatment of anal carcinoma.

Surg Oncol Clin N Am 26 (2017) xiii–xiv
http://dx.doi.org/10.1016/j.soc.2016.08.001
1055-3207/17/© 2016 Published by Elsevier Inc.

I would like to thank Dr Cathy Eng for pulling together an outstanding group of individuals with expertise in this disease site.

Nicholas J. Petrelli, MD, FACS
Helen F. Graham Cancer Center
& Research Institute
Christiana Care Health Systems
4701 Ogletown-Stanton Road, Suite 1233
Newark, DE 19713, USA

E-mail address:
npetrelli@christianacare.org

Preface

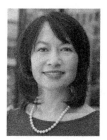

Cathy Eng, MD, FACP
Editor

Carcinoma of the anal canal is a malignancy that has been underrecognized for several years largely due to its low incidence relative to other gastrointestinal cancers. Anal cancer may also be of lesser interest since the majority of patients will present with locally advanced disease and are treated with a standard regimen of combined concurrent chemoradiation therapy. This approach has remained unchanged for 4 decades. Due to the low incidence of anal cancer in the United States, it was likely a practicing physician would only evaluate and treat less than 10 patients per year. Yet, the incidence of anal cancer continues to rise annually over the past decade; more than 8,000 individuals in the United States annually will be diagnosed with anal cancer. Globally, it is estimated more than 27,000 individuals are diagnosed with anal cancer annually. Furthermore, the association of the human papilloma virus (HPV) and the development of anal carcinoma as well as other HPV-associated malignancies, such as cervical and oropharyngeal cancer, is well established. Hence, there has been a resurgence of academic interest in this patient population.

In this issue of *Surgical Oncology Clinics of North America*, we have gathered a multidisciplinary group of internationally renowned experts to provide their expertise on various topics of interest, including epidemiology, pathogenesis, the impact of immunocompromised states and the development of anal cancer, treatment of anal dysplasia, as well as approaches to locally advanced, recurrent, and metastatic disease. Other articles of interest include radiation therapy as well as an article dedicated to rare non–squamous cell anal carcinoma subtypes.

With the continued rise in anal carcinoma, physicians will need to be more familiar with treating this malignancy in order to optimize patient care and outcome. Given the extensive expertise from my coauthors, we hope this focused issue of *Surgical*

Surg Oncol Clin N Am 26 (2017) xv–xvi
http://dx.doi.org/10.1016/j.soc.2016.09.001
1055-3207/17/© 2016 Published by Elsevier Inc.

surgonc.theclinics.com

Oncology Clinics of North America on anal cancer will serve as a valuable resource for all practicing physicians.

Cathy Eng, MD, FACP
Colorectal Center
The University of Texas M.D. Anderson Cancer Center
Department of Gastrointestinal Medical Oncology
1515 Holcombe Boulevard, Unit 426
Houston, TX 77030, USA

E-mail address:
ceng@mdanderson.org

Patient Perspective and Personal Journey of Treating a "Rare Cancer"

Michele Longabaugh, RN

KEYWORDS

- Anal cancer • Anal cancer awareness • Anal cancer support • HPV vaccination

KEY POINTS

- The diagnosis of advanced stage anal cancer requires facing the challenges posed, including the search for expert care and the personal road to achieving a "no evidence of disease state."
- There are difficulties in raising awareness of early detection for rare cancers, including care provider education for recognition and screening, and general population education.
- Researchers and pharmaceutical companies have refocused on improving treatment options for patients, especially those in the advanced stages of anal cancer.
- The lack of available resources must be recognized. Health care tools, support, and advocacy for the anal cancer community must be found.
- Topnotch care through networking support between larger and local cancer care centers must be provided. Prevention must be promoted through immunization and ending unwarranted stigma.

PERSONAL STORY: ANAL CANCER, ONLY "RARE" TO THOSE WHO DO NOT HAVE IT

I heard the words "you have cancer" just a few days after my 47th birthday. As shocking as those words are to the thousands that hear them each year, nothing on earth could prepare me for the statement that followed, "It's anal cancer, stage IV." How could this be? Up until that day I had been living an average and fulfilling life for a middle-aged female. I was happily married for 23 years, enjoyed my life as a wife and mother of 3, worked as a registered nurse, and was in good health and good shape. I am a nonsmoker, no history of known human papillomavirus (HPV) or positive Papanicolaou (Pap) smears. I always complied with yearly visits for well-woman assessment and mammography. And, aside from symptoms of recurrent anal itching and bleeding, which I regarded as a hemorrhoid, and my chronic sciatica,

Disclosure Statement: The author has nothing to disclose.
BIOTRONIK Inc., Saleswest Field Support, 6024 Jean Road, Lake Oswego, OR 97035, USA
E-mail address: michele.longabaugh@att.net

I was a typical Midwestern woman. That day in 2010 changed my life in ways I could never fathom.

My road to diagnosis began back in July of 2009 with what I thought was a fairly routine hemorrhoid flare up. I had struggled with them intermittently for about 16 years since the birth of my last child. This attack never really cleared up and I continued to treat it with over-the-counter medicines for several months. It was not until I started actively bleeding into the toilet and the itching became unbearable that I decided I must consult with a physician even though it felt embarrassing and awkward. I delayed this 2 additional months because my yearly gynecologic examination was scheduled for early January. I felt the least self-conscious with this physician, most likely due to the nature of the examination. This experience is not unique for anal cancer patients with my demographics. I dismissed symptoms for months, not realizing the life-threatening consequences of this 6-month delay. My gynecologist (GYN) was quick to recognize there was a problem when I complained about my hemorrhoid at that annual well-woman examination and asked him to check it for me. The color literally drained from his face when he was examining me and he saw the skin lesion. He had never seen anything like it before and did not know what it was. I was swab tested for a yeast infection and was immediately referred to a colorectal surgeon (CRS). I inquired about my increasing sciatica and he suggested that I follow up with my primary care physician (PCP) in regard to the pain. The next week I was examined by a CRS and he was also unclear about what the skin lesion was. He performed 3 biopsies under local anesthesia in the office that day. At that time, I again mentioned my sciatic pain and he concurred with my GYN and referred me back to my PCP to address it. My CRS diagnosed me with high-grade anal intraepithelial neoplasia (AIN) 3 days later, a colonoscopy was scheduled for the next week, and I was pre-scribed 5-fluorouracil (FU) cream.

Anxious to learn all I could about my diagnosis, the Internet seemed like a good place to start. Information and data available on AIN were scarce, and what was available was technical and frightening. The more I learned about it the more I came to understand that I was battling more than simply a rare form of carcinoma in situ. There is a stigma attached to this disease. The stigma of anal cancer can be paralyzing. The isolation is notable. However, as a health care professional, I was undaunted. I began a search for support, and reliable and relevant information about my currently prescribed treatment.

On further exploration by my PCP via MRI the following week, my continued sciatica was determined to be caused by a large lesion growing out of my sacral L1 vertebrae and compressing the nerve. This became the catalyst for my anal cancer diagnosis. I was referred to a neurosurgeon. In the meantime, the colonoscopy was done and, aside from seeing "much of the same" type of lesion just inside the entrance of my anus, which was also biopsied, the results were unremarkable and no further testing was recommended. I was instructed to continue with the 5-FU cream. I saw the neurosurgeon a few days later to discuss the tumor in my sacrum. A computed tomography (CT) scan was immediately scheduled, with surgery to follow. At first, there was significant doubt about any correlation with AIN. I even asked specifically if the tumor in my sacrum could be related to the AIN and both the CRS and neurosurgeon were dubious about whether the 2 were related. The neurosurgeon did not immediately recognize the type of cancer cells. An oncologist was consulted. The pathologist, together with my oncologist, finally fit all the pieces together. I had poorly differentiated stage IV anal canal carcinoma. I had 2 tumors at my anal opening with bone metastasis to my sacrum. A PET scan revealed no other distance sites. My prognosis was poor. I underwent treatment at my local cancer center. I received the standard Nigro protocol, with

4 additional sites added to the pelvic radiation. I spent the last 2 weeks of treatment in the hospital for pain control and management of burns due to a hyper-response to radiation. I survived and a surprising 2 years of disease-free state followed, confirmed by CT scans every 90 days. My sciatica returned in September 2012 and that prompted a PET scan follow-up that revealed a lesion in the lateral lower lobe of my right lung. After 30 days, upon repeat imaging, it showed growth and was determined to be suspicious enough to warrant removal. I underwent thoracotomy with a wedge resection of the lesion and the placement of gold seeds for future robotic radiosurgery use if needed. It was determined by pathologic evaluation to be poorly differentiated squamous cell carcinoma. Clean margins were obtained, so no further treatment was indicated. Close surveillance followed and 2 other lung lesions became active 6 months later, this time in the hilar region of the right lower lobe confirmed to be squamous cell carcinoma by biopsy. I was then referred for care to the University of Texas MD Anderson Cancer Center. After consultation, I underwent 4 rounds of chemotherapy, cisplatin with 5-FU, followed by 2 weeks of targeted radiation to the area. There has been no evidence of disease since October 2013. Although my story in itself is not unusual, my outcome has been nothing short of miraculous.

CARE PROVIDERS: AWARENESS, PREVENTION, AND TREATMENT

Many rare cancers are limited by lack of medical (education or treatment) infrastructure. My cancer was not readily recognized. Solutions must be found to facilitate caregiver education about rare cancers and their correlating symptoms. Early detection is crucial to positive outcomes. Wide-scale awareness of anal cancer has to be addressed for both the general population and medical community. My lack of general lower gastrointestinal (GI) cancer symptom awareness contributed greatly to my delay in diagnosis. This extended to my health care provider as well. When patients present to their PCP with complaints of a hemorrhoid, the examination needs to go beyond prescription-strength hemorrhoid pharmaceuticals. Digital rectal examination and anal pap smears need to become the standard of care for patients presenting with hemorrhoid symptoms.

Although standard-of-care initiatives are vital, actually getting the population to overcome the embarrassment to start the conversation with their primary health care providers is a hurdle that must be addressed. Long-term bleeding, itching, and hemorrhoid treatment is a recurrent theme among anal cancer victims. Even as a registered nurse, I failed to recognize these symptoms as anything other than benign and, even when they persisted and I became suspicious, awkwardness held me back from seeking treatment more promptly. Had I not had been scheduled for my annual gynecologic examination and PAP smear, it might have remained unaddressed for a few more months. Truly, it was the sciatica that really uncovered the identity of the anal cancer. I had been misdiagnosed with AIN just a few weeks before the MRI, which was prompted by my unrelenting sciatica. Nobody was looking for anal cancer.

How should this be addressed? Large-scale education is required for the increased prevalence of this cancer and could be included with other HPV-related cancer education. Family practice, internal medicine, obstetrics (OB), and GYN physicians need to be properly educated to be on the lookout for anal cancer. It starts with the standard of care for the patient complaining of persistent hemorrhoids, rectal bleeding, and/or itching. Office materials, brochures, and posters in waiting areas and treatment rooms of clinics could prove beneficial. Widespread public service announcements would reach more people in vulnerable populations. I failed to recognize that my first screening room was my bathroom. Had I understood that rectal bleeding and itching for longer than a week could be indicative of a more serious underlying problem and required a more comprehensive examination, I would have sought treatment months before. I thought I had a hemorrhoid and was simply embarrassed to seek examination. These symptoms are shared with other lower GI cancers, which also suffer the same "awkward" location. That being said, anal cancer is treated by the same specialists for surgical intervention and oncology. A call from the medical community to initiate a large-scale awareness campaign that includes all lower GI cancers could create tremendous impact in the early detection of colon, rectal, and anal cancer.

A medical care provider hurdle that accompanies the diagnosis of anal canal carcinoma is finding reliable, understandable information regarding treatment and care. Rare cancers lack the typical medical information scaffolding that more common disease states (eg, breast cancer) possess. There are forums, Web sites, and data centers available for more prevalent cancers. This networking integrates the medical community with the patient population and reliable information is easily and readily available to those who seek it. It is typically offered, unsolicited, as part of the care of these patients. Not so with anal cancer. In 2010, I was only able to find a handful of small technical studies, all related to HPV or human immunodeficiency virus (HIV). Because only a few patients in my community were diagnosed each year, my caregivers lacked the resources that are crucial to optimal outcomes for anal cancer patients.

The importance of provider experience is critical for management of short-term side effects as a result of treatment, as well as for the potential long-term side effects that anal cancer survivors experience. I wish I had been treated like I was going to survive from the start of my treatments.

In the short term, nausea, vomiting, dehydration, unrelenting diarrhea, pain with urination, and burns were treated as they arose. The same strategy of "wait and see" seems common for long-term side-effect management. Once I recovered from the initial insult of therapy, the long-term side effects of radiation exposure began within a few months. Pelvic floor dysfunction effected my ability to hold my urine or my stool in the case of diarrhea, allow a bowel movement under normal conditions, or to resume sexual intercourse. I am plagued by symptoms brought on by early onset menopause. I struggle with nutrition. All of the long-term effects previously discussed were addressed after they occurred. Ongoing palliative care is essential to mitigation and/or prevention of the known and the unknown long-term effects of pelvic radiation and must be part of the care plan for the anal cancer patient.

Change is needed in regard to the treatment and care of the anal cancer patient. Aside from the treatment protocol that has essentially not been altered in more than 30 years, the overall care could be markedly improved. Anal cancer, as most rare cancers, is a challenge to manage simply because of lack of experience with such patients. Lack of large-scale organizations that offer support to these patients and their caregivers leaves a gaping hole that for other cancers (eg, breast cancer) is easily filled. The treatment regime for anal cancer is brutal because it involves simultaneous chemotherapy and pelvic radiation. Understanding the short-term and long-term treatment challenges and side effects facing the anal cancer patient is important. Knowledge is power; therefore, helping to educate patients and caregivers on what to expect and what the plan of action will be when the side effects occur will benefit all involved. This goes far beyond the nausea and vomiting that chemotherapy brings. It extends to skin care for radiation burns; bladder and bowel control for before, during, and after treatments have concluded; diet intolerance and nutrition; pain management; and sexual dysfunction. Proactive intervention is critical in maximizing the recovery of the patient and ensuring maximum quality of life (QOL). Pelvic floor physical therapy plays a vital role in optimal recovery for patients early after anal cancer treatments have concluded. This requires long-term palliative support for the patient. Sexual counseling and therapy need to be prescribed at the onset and throughout treatment and recovery. This should be presented as a long-term expectation.

When I bring up my side effects, it is often expressed to me that I should simply be happy to be alive. This attitude is prevalent in both my personal life and the health care community. QOL is a vital part of human existence. Patients with rare cancers receive very little attention regarding the QOL experienced during and after treatment. Palliative care could play an essential role in minimizing these side effects (eg, pelvic floor physical therapy during and after treatment, use of vaginal dilators during radiation treatment, topical vaginal hormone therapy, and counseling for sexual dysfunction). QOL surveys are an essential tool for helping to determine the patient needs.

RESEARCH: IMPROVING TREATMENT OPTIONS

Research to advance and improve the treatment and outcomes for anal cancer patients is needed. Many pharmaceutical companies turned from exploring alternative or new anal cancer treatment regimens to focus on the HPV vaccine when they discovered that immunization would significantly decrease anal cancer incidence. Who could foresee the poor acceptance of this vaccination? According to the President's Cancer Panel's report on HPV vaccination, only one-third of eligible 13 to 17-year-old girls had completed the 3-vaccine series and less than 7% of their male peers had done so in 2012. This is due, in part, to the later approval of males to receive the vaccine (2006 for girls vs 2011 for boys); however, the rates of vaccinated boys are still lower than those observed for girls at a comparable time after approval[1] (**Fig. 1**).

Again, vaccination acceptance is directly affected by the stigma of a sexually transmitted disease. The numbers of squamous cell carcinoma cases continues to rise at a

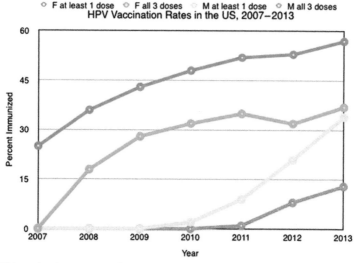

Fig. 1. HPV vaccination rates in the US are improving but are still not sufficient, especially among the male population. F, female patients; M, male patients.

somewhat alarming rate. The American Cancer Society estimates for anal cancer in the United States for 2016 are about 8080 new cases (5160 in women and 2920 in men) and about 1080 deaths (640 in women and 440 in men).

The number of new anal cancer cases has been rising for many years. Anal cancer is rare in people younger than 35 years and is found mainly in older adults, with the average age in the early 60s.[2]

Researchers and drug companies must refocus to provide options for improved and effective treatment opportunities, especially for advanced stages of the disease. Options remain limited and those that do exist are difficult to access due to the rare nature of anal cancer. The participation rate in clinical trials overall is less than 5%. Murthy and colleagues[3] calculated an enrollment rate of 1.7% in clinical trials sponsored by the National Cancer Institute when divided by the total estimated cancer cases in the United States. Eng and colleagues[4] concluded that, with only a 0.65% enrollment (Al-Refaie and colleagues[5]) among 244,528 of subjects (with melanoma, breast, lung, esophagus, gastric, liver, pancreas, colon, rectum, or anal cancers) in the California Registry between 2001 and 2008, ways must be found to increase access, improve design, and speed completion of clinical trials. From a patient perspective, access to clinical trials for patients with any type of cancer, common or rare, primary or recurrent, is vital.

THE CHALLENGE: BUILDING SUPPORT

The quandary for the patient with a rare cancer is the lack of available resources. Finding health care tools and advocacy is a fundamental struggle. When faced with more common cancers, resources are easily accessible. There is no lack of community when one is diagnosed with breast or prostate cancer. The patient is buoyed by a well-organized community with resources often offered directly within the oncology clinic itself. Education, support groups, Web sites, study availability, and the resources to help navigate these tools are readily available. Not so for those diagnosed with anal cancer. Especially for those at a distance from large centers. The patient must initiate their own search for resources and create their own community of support. With such an overwhelming, stigmatized, and squeamish type of diagnosis, patients are often relegated to silence. Isolation is a frequent side effect of anal cancer. This isolation perpetuates the problem of finding broad support for this orphan cancer.

Even large cancer organizations offer little for the patient with rare cancer. Since my diagnosis in 2010, the HPV and Anal Cancer Foundation[6] has been founded in New York City, offering reliable medical information and resources, as well as an active peer-to-peer program. This foundation is a leader on the anal cancer front. Necessity, being the natural mother of invention, has forced self-advocacy among patients. Smaller Web sites started by patients with rare cancers exist and virtual support groups facilitated by patients in many social media forums have been created to help assist those afflicted and affected by anal cancer to find each other.

SOLUTIONS: WHAT CAN BE DONE?

The solutions are not simple but they are attainable. Patients are leading the way by demanding care and demanding change. Knowledge is power for physicians and the general population. It is imperative the medical community (eg, CRSs, OB/GYNs, PCPs, and pediatricians) be educated in screening and prevention. Immunization is the key to reducing incidence of anal cancer for future generations. Networking support between larger cancer care centers and community-based cancer care centers is vital when providing treatment of anal cancer patients. Ongoing palliative care can help in the management and QOL of patients with anal cancer or other rare cancers. Helping patients, their families, and caregivers to seek out support and research opportunities is an essential part of the complete care of the patient. Finally, the accompanying stigma associated with anal cancer cannot be discounted for its impact on patient experience and overall treatment. There is no room for blame in cancer care. Although I was always overtly treated with dignity and respect, there was an underlying sense of judgment. I felt the stigma associated with my HPV-related cancer from family, friends, and health care providers alike. I felt responsible for somehow causing my cancer. Patients do not deserve the judgment placed on them by others. The responsibility of erasing stigma starts with the health care community. They must lead the way to end the unwarranted shame of an anal cancer diagnosis. It is the gateway to prevention, awareness, early diagnosis, and successful treatment of anal cancer.

REFERENCES

1. President's Cancer Panel annual report executive summary accelerating HPV vaccine uptake 2012-2013. Available at: http://deainfo.nci.nih.gov/advisory/pcp/annualReports/HPV/ExecutiveSummary.htm#sthash.LR9ZMtQt.dpbs. Accessed March 10, 2016.
2. American Cancer Society key statistics for anal cancer. Available at: http://www.cancer.org/cancer/analcancer/detailedguide/anal-cancer-what-is-key-statistics. Accessed March 12, 2016.
3. Murthy VH, Krumholz HM, Gross CP. Participation in cancer clinical trials: race-, sex-, and age based disparities. JAMA 2004;291:2720–6.
4. Eng C, Roach N, Longabaugh M, et al. Perspectives on clinical trials for gastrointestinal malignancies. Am Soc Clin Oncol Educ Book 2015;40–3. Available at: asco.org/edbook.
5. Al-Refaie WB, Vickers SM, Zhong W, et al. Cancer trials versus the real world in the United States. Ann Surg 2011;254:438–42.
6. HPV and Anal Cancer Foundation connect with a peer. Available at: http://www.analcancerfoundation.org/find-support/patient-support/connect-with-a-peer/. Accessed February 20, 2016.

Epidemiology of Anal Canal Cancer

Valerie M. Nelson, MD, MBA, Al B. Benson III, MD*

KEYWORDS

• Anal canal • Epidemiology • HPV • HIV

KEY POINTS

• Anal canal cancer is a rare malignancy.
• The incidence of anal canal cancer is increasing, particularly among young men.
• Risk factors for anal cancer include human papilloma virus (HPV) infection, human immunodeficiency virus (HIV) infection, more than 10 sexual partners, and anoreceptive intercourse.
• Anal cancer risk increases with the duration of HIV infection.
• The increased incidence in anal cancer is caused by increased prevalence of HPV and longer survival of individuals infected with HIV.

INTRODUCTION

Anal cancer is an uncommon malignancy, but the incidence of this disease has been increasing over the past 30 years. This article focuses on anal canal squamous cell cancers (SCCAs), which comprise most anal canal cancers. Risk factors for anal canal cancer are well established, including human papillomavirus (HPV) infection and human immunodeficiency virus (HIV) infection, both of which correlate with increased number of sexual partners and anoreceptive intercourse. The increase in anal cancer is attributed to multiple factors, including increased prevalence of HPV and longer survival of individuals infected with HIV.

OVERVIEW

Anal canal cancer refers to malignancy of the mucosa-lined anal canal arising from 1 to 2 cm proximal to the dentate line to the intersphincteric groove separating the anal margin from the anal canal.[1] Roughly 85% of anal canal cancers are of squamous cell origin.[2] Of the remaining cases, roughly 10% are adenocarcinoma and 5% are

Disclosure: The authors have nothing to disclose.
Hematology/Oncology, Department of Medicine, Robert H. Lurie Comprehensive Cancer Center, Feinberg School of Medicine, Northwestern University, 676 N Saint Clair, Suite 850, Chicago, IL 60611, USA
* Corresponding author.
E-mail address: a-benson@northwestern.edu

rare tumor types such as melanoma, small cell carcinoma, and tumors metastatic from other sites.[3]

The American Cancer Society estimates there will be 8080 new cases of anal (anus, anal canal, and anorectum) cancer in 2016, roughly 60% of which will be in women.[4] It is estimated that 1080 individuals will die from their disease. Although generally considered a rare cancer, representing 2.7% of all digestive malignancies and less than 0.5% of all diagnosed malignancies, the incidence of SCCA has been increasing over the last few decades.[2,4]

RISK FACTORS
Sexual Activity

Risk factors for anal cancer were initially determined by case-control studies comparing men and women with anal cancer with normal control subjects and patients with adenocarcinoma of the colon or rectum. For example, Frisch and colleagues[5] compared 417 patients with anal cancer with 534 patients with adenocarcinoma of the rectum and 554 normal control subjects. The relative risk of anal cancer was highest in people with 10 or more sexual partners or history of sexually transmitted diseases (STDs) such as HIV, herpes, gonorrhea, syphilis, and chlamydia (**Box 1**).[5]

Human Papilloma Virus

As noted earlier, sexual activity was found to be a risk factor for anal cancer. In addition, an increased risk of anal cancer was noted in individuals with cervical cancer. As the link between cervical cancer and HPV became established, investigators speculated that HPV might also be causative in anal cancer. The well-established progression from HPV infection to cervical intraepithelial neoplasia to cervical malignancy led to exploration of anal epithelial neoplasia as a precursor lesion to SCCA.[6]

Increasing evidence indicates that the oncogenic strains of HPV, specifically subtypes 16 and 18, cause SCCA in the anal canal as they are known to do in the cervix and head and neck.[7–9] Early evidence, including a study by Frisch and colleagues,[5] that found HPV DNA in 88% of patients with anal cancer but in none of the patients with rectal cancer in the series. HPV subtype 16 was involved in 73% of the anal cancer cases.[5]

HPV risk factors include increased number of sexual partners, anoreceptive intercourse, and other STDs, particularly underlying HIV infection.[10,11] Thus many of the

---

Box 1
Risk factors for anal canal cancer

HPV infection

HIV infection

More than 10 lifetime sexual partners

Anoreceptive intercourse

Chronic immunosuppression

Cigarette smoking

History of gynecologic or hematologic malignancy

early identified sexual risk factors are simply risks for acquisition of oncogenic HPV strains.[12] Not surprisingly, personal history of one HPV-associated malignancy is a risk factor to acquire a second HPV-associated malignancy.[13]

The prevalence of HPV in the United States is variable, ranging from 10% in low-risk groups to nearly 90% in individuals infected with HIV.[14-16] It is thought that HPV is associated with 65% to 89% of all SCCA of the anal canal, making this the leading risk factor for this malignancy.[17,18] A recent series of 72 metastatic anal cancer cases at MD Anderson revealed that 94% had detectable HPV.[19] Note that, unlike in head and neck cancer, in which HPV-positive disease portends improved prognosis, the prognostic value of HPV in anal cancer is unknown.[20]

Human Immunodeficiency Virus

HIV infection is a well-established risk factor for anal canal cancer. However, the risk of SCCA is not reduced by the use of highly active antiretroviral therapy (HAART).[21] Some degree of the increased incidence of anal cancer in general is likely caused by improvements in HIV patient survival because the risk for SCCA increases with the duration of HIV infection; there is a 12-fold greater risk of anal cancer for persons who have been infected with HIV for 15 years or longer compared with those who have been infected with HIV for 5 years or less.[22,23] The increased incidence in anal canal cancer from 19.0 per 100,000 person-years from 1992 to 1995 to 78.2 per 100,000 person-years from 2000 to 2003 correlates with the natural history of HIV and HPV coinfections starting during the HIV epidemic in the 1980s.[24] Specifically, the expected progression from viral infection to HPV-associated anal epithelial changes to development of SCCA would be expected to take 1 to 2 decades.[25]

Chronic Immunosuppression

It is well established that anal cancer occurs at increased rates in patients with chronic immunosuppression either because of inherited or acquired immunodeficiency.[3] For example, there is a 10-fold to 100-fold increased relative risk for SCCA in renal transplant patients.[26,27] Some of this risk is mediated by HPV infections because the infection rate in new renal transplant patients is 23% but increases to 47% in established renal transplant patients.[26,27] Similarly there is a 4-fold increased relative risk for SCCA in cardiac transplant patients.[28]

Other types of immunosuppression, such as chronic steroid use or immunomodulators used for treatment of autoimmune diseases, are not as clearly linked to SCCA, although there is an increased likelihood of persistent HPV infection.[29]

There is some evidence of increased risk of HPV-driven cervical cancer in patients with inflammatory bowel disease,[30] but no definitively increased risk has been shown for anal cancer in these patients.[31]

Tobacco Use

Case-control studies indicate that cigarette smoking significantly increases the risk of contracting anal cancer.[19,32,33] There seems to be a direct correlation between number of cigarettes smoked and increased relative risk. Specifically, Holly and colleagues[32] found a relative risk of 1.9 for persons with a 20-pack-year smoking history and a relative risk of 5.2 for persons with a 50-pack-year history. Current smoking is the highest risk, with a relative risk of 7.7 in women and 9.4 in men.[12]

INCREASING INCIDENCE, CHANGING DEMOGRAPHICS

A Surveillance, Epidemiology, and End Results (SEER) database review of data from 1973 to 2009 showed that incidence rates of SCCA increased dramatically after 1997.[25] This higher incidence has been attributed to 2 major factors. First, successful use of HAART has resulted in longer survival of individuals with HIV infection, which increases SCCA risk over time. Second, an increase in high risk sexual activity resulted in increased HPV acquisition rates.[25]

In the period from 1997 to 2009, the annual percentage change in incidence of anal canal cancers (including carcinoma in situ) was 7.2%. The annual percentage change was 9.5% in men and 4.5% in women, with growth most prevalent in men aged less than 65 years.[25] Recent data indicate that anal cancer is most common in men aged 35 to 49 years followed by those aged 50 to 64 years, whereas for women the most common age range is age greater than or equal to 65 years followed by ages 50 to 64 years.[25] The increased risk was consistent across ethnic groups with the exception of Hispanic white women, who experienced a less prominently increased risk.[25]

HUMAN PAPILLOMA VIRUS VACCINE

Given that most SCCA is caused by the HPV virus, there is much enthusiasm surrounding the use of HPV vaccines as a cancer prevention tool. There are 3 commercially available HPV vaccines, as shown in **Table 1**. When given to appropriate patient populations, the vaccines are expected to reduce rates of many gynecologic cancers, anal cancer, and head and neck cancer. Although efficacy data regarding reduction of anal cancer rates are not yet available, surrogate markers indicate that this approach holds promise. For example, a study of women who participated in a bivalent vaccine trial showed 84% risk reduction in the acquisition of HPV types 16 and 18 in the anus.[34] In a planned substudy of 604 men who have sex with men (MSM), the quadrivalent vaccine was shown to prevent the development of intraepithelial neoplasia caused by HPV in 78% of previously HPV-naive men.[35] The United States Advisory Committee on Immunization Practices (ACIP) recommends the quadrivalent or 9-valent HPV vaccine for the prevention of anal cancer in women.[36] The ACIP also recommends vaccination of MSM who are at high risk for HPV infection.[36]

In the United States, vaccine underuse has been an ongoing concern. A 2012 report estimated that vaccine coverage among teenage girls was 54% for 1 dose and only 33% for the recommend 3 doses.[37] Reasons cited for poor vaccine penetrance include lack of knowledge about vaccine benefits, concerns about vaccine safety, and parental perception that their children were not sexually active and therefore did not need to be vaccinated.[37] Increased HPV vaccine use by young adults may be the most cost-effective mechanism to prevent morbidity and mortality from SCCA in the coming decades.[38]

Table 1 HPV vaccines, HPV types included, and administration		
Vaccine	HPV Type	Administration Intervals (mo)
Quadrivalent (Gardasil)	6, 11, 16, 18	0, 2, and 6
9-Valent (Gardasil 9)	6, 11, 16, 18, 31, 33, 45, 52, 58	0, 2, and 6
Bivalent (Cervarix)	16, 18	0, 1, 6

SUMMARY

In summary, although anal canal cancer remains an uncommon malignancy, the incidence is increasing in recent decades, particularly in young men. The most common cause of anal cancer is HPV infection, particularly subtypes 16 and 18, and with patients with HIV/HPV coinfection are at particularly increased risk. Many behavioral risk factors, such as increased number of sexual partners and anoreceptive intercourse, are mediated through HPV infection acquisition. Important nonsexual risk factors include chronic immunosuppression and cigarette smoking. It remains to be seen how the HPV vaccine will affect the incidence of anal canal cancer in coming decades.

REFERENCES

1. Edge SB, Byrd DR, Compton CC, et al. AJCC cancer staging manual. 7th edition. New York: Springer; 2010.
2. Johnson LG, Madeleine MM, Newcomer LM, et al. Anal cancer incidence and survival: the surveillance, epidemiology, and end results experience, 1973-2000. Cancer 2004;101(2):281–8.
3. Longacre TA, Kong CS, Welton ML. Diagnostic problems in anal pathology. Adv Anat Pathol 2008;15(5):263–78.
4. Siegel RL, Miller KD, Jemal A. Cancer statistics, 2016. CA Cancer J Clin 2016; 66(1):7–30.
5. Frisch M, Glimelius B, van den Brule AJ, et al. Sexually transmitted infection as a cause of anal cancer. N Engl J Med 1997;337(19):1350–8.
6. Fenger C. Anal neoplasia and its precursors: facts and controversies. Semin Diagn Pathol 1991;8(3):190–201.
7. Palefsky J. Human papillomavirus and anal neoplasia. Curr HIV/AIDS Rep 2008; 5(2):78–85.
8. Gravitt PE. The known unknowns of HPV natural history. J Clin Invest 2011; 121(12):4593–9.
9. Gillison ML, Koch WM, Capone RB, et al. Evidence for a causal association between human papillomavirus and a subset of head and neck cancers. J Natl Cancer Inst 2000;92(9):709–20.
10. Machalek DA, Poynten M, Jin F, et al. Anal human papillomavirus infection and associated neoplastic lesions in men who have sex with men: a systematic review and meta-analysis. Lancet Oncol 2012;13(5):487–500.
11. Hariri S, Unger ER, Sternberg M, et al. Prevalence of genital human papillomavirus among females in the United States, the National Health and Nutrition Examination Survey, 2003-2006. J Infect Dis 2011;204(4):566–73.
12. Daling JR, Weiss NS, Hislop TG, et al. Sexual practices, sexually transmitted diseases, and the incidence of anal cancer. N Engl J Med 1987;317(16):973–7.
13. Frisch M, Olsen JH, Melbye M. Malignancies that occur before and after anal cancer: clues to their etiology. Am J Epidemiol 1994;140(1):12–9.
14. Gaffga NH, Flagg EW, Weinstock HS, et al. Monitoring HPV type-specific prevalence over time through clinic-based surveillance: a perspective on vaccine effectiveness. Vaccine 2012;30(11):1959–64.
15. Palefsky JM, Holly EA, Ralston ML, et al. Prevalence and risk factors for anal human papillomavirus infection in human immunodeficiency virus (HIV)-positive and high-risk HIV-negative women. J Infect Dis 2001;183(3):383–91.
16. Palefsky JM, Holly EA, Ralston ML, et al. Prevalence and risk factors for human papillomavirus infection of the anal canal in human immunodeficiency virus

(HIV)-positive and HIV-negative homosexual men. J Infect Dis 1998;177(2): 361–7.

17. Frisch M, Fenger C, van den Brule AJ, et al. Variants of squamous cell carcinoma of the anal canal and perianal skin and their relation to human papillomaviruses. Cancer Res 1999;59(3):753–7.

18. Melbye M, Frisch M. The role of human papillomaviruses in anogenital cancers. Semin Cancer Biol 1998;8(4):307–13.

19. Morris VK, Rashid A, Rodriguez-Bigas M, et al. Clinicopathologic features associated with human papillomavirus/p16 in patients with metastatic squamous cell carcinoma of the anal canal. Oncologist 2015;20(11):1247–52.

20. Williams GR, Lu QL, Love SB, et al. Properties of HPV-positive and HPV-negative anal carcinomas. J Pathol 1996;180(4):378–82.

21. Lim ST, Levine AM. Non-AIDS-defining cancers and HIV infection. Curr Infect Dis Rep 2005;7(3):227–34.

22. Crum-Cianflone NF, Hullsiek KH, Marconi VC, et al. Anal cancers among HIV-infected persons: HAART is not slowing rising incidence. AIDS 2010;24(4): 535–43.

23. Palefsky JM, Holly EA, Efirdc JT, et al. Anal intraepithelial neoplasia in the highly active antiretroviral therapy era among HIV-positive men who have sex with men. AIDS 2005;19(13):1407–14.

24. Patel P, Hanson DL, Sullivan PS, et al. Incidence of types of cancer among HIV-infected persons compared with the general population in the United States, 1992-2003. Ann Intern Med 2008;148(10):728–36.

25. Nelson RA, Levine AM, Bernstein L, et al. Changing patterns of anal canal carcinoma in the United States. J Clin Oncol 2013;31(12):1569–75.

26. Patel HS, Silver AR, Northover JM. Anal cancer in renal transplant patients. Int J Colorectal Dis 2007;22(1):1–5.

27. Arends MJ, Benton EC, McLaren KM, et al. Renal allograft recipients with high susceptibility to cutaneous malignancy have an increased prevalence of human papillomavirus DNA in skin tumours and a greater risk of anogenital malignancy. Br J Cancer 1997;75(5):722–8.

28. Chapman JR, Webster AC, Wong G. Cancer in the transplant recipient. Cold Spring Harb Perspect Med 2013;3(7):a015677.

29. Sillman FH, Sedlis A. Anogenital papillomavirus infection and neoplasia in immunodeficient women: an update. Dermatol Clin 1991;9(2):353–69.

30. Bhatia J, Bratcher J, Korelitz B, et al. Abnormalities of uterine cervix in women with inflammatory bowel disease. World J Gastroenterol 2006;12(38):6167–71.

31. Frisch M, Olsen JH, Bautz A, et al. Benign anal lesions and the risk of anal cancer. N Engl J Med 1994;331(5):300–2.

32. Holly EA, Whittemore AS, Aston DA, et al. Anal cancer incidence: genital warts, anal fissure or fistula, hemorrhoids, and smoking. J Natl Cancer Inst 1989; 81(22):1726–31.

33. Bertisch B, Franceschi S, Lise M, et al. Risk factors for anal cancer in persons infected with HIV: a nested case-control study in the Swiss HIV Cohort Study. Am J Epidemiol 2013;178(6):877–84.

34. Kreimer AR, Gonzalez P, Katki HA, et al. Efficacy of a bivalent HPV 16/18 vaccine against anal HPV 16/18 infection among young women: a nested analysis within the Costa Rica Vaccine Trial. Lancet Oncol 2011;12(9):862–70.

35. Giuliano AR, Palefsky JM, Goldstone S, et al. Efficacy of quadrivalent HPV vaccine against HPV Infection and disease in males. N Engl J Med 2011;364(5): 401–11.

36. Markowitz LE, Dunne EF, Saraiya M, et al. Human papillomavirus vaccination: recommendations of the Advisory Committee on Immunization Practices (ACIP). MMWR Recomm Rep 2014;63(RR-05):1–30.
37. Centers for Disease Cancer Prevention. Human papillomavirus vaccination coverage among adolescent girls, 2007-2012, and postlicensure vaccine safety monitoring, 2006-2013 – United States. MMWR Morb Mortal Wkly Rep 2013; 62(29):591–5.
38. Sanders GD, Taira AV. Cost-effectiveness of a potential vaccine for human papillomavirus. Emerg Infect Dis 2003;9(1):37–48.

Human Immunodeficiency Virus/AIDS, Human Papillomavirus, and Anal Cancer

CrossMark

Chia-ching J. Wang, MD[a], Joseph Sparano, MD[b],
Joel M. Palefsky, MD[c],*

KEYWORDS

• HPV • HPV vaccination • Anal cancer • HIV • Immunosuppression

KEY POINTS

• Anal cancer is preceded by precursor lesions; it is also almost always associated with human papillomavirus (HPV) infection.

• The degree to which highly active antiretroviral therapy (HAART) prevents the development or progression of anal high-grade squamous intraepithelial lesions (HSIL) to anal cancer is not known.

• Both HPV infection and anal HSIL clearly occur in individuals well-controlled on HAART; overall the incidence of anal cancer is higher in the HAART era than the pre-HAART era.

• Individuals infected with human immunodeficiency virus (HIV) who have anal cancer can receive similar treatment as HIV-negative individuals and achieve similar outcomes, but may require careful monitoring for toxicities.

• The use of a screening anal cytology in high-risk patients may lead to an earlier diagnosis of anal HSIL, and treatment of HSIL may decrease the risk for developing anal cancer.

INTRODUCTION

Human papillomavirus (HPV), the most common sexually transmitted infection worldwide, causes approximately 5% of all cancers in men and 10% of all cancers in women.[1] Anal cancer is highly associated with HPV infection. Similar to cervical

Disclosure Statement: Dr J.M. Palefsky is a member of a Merck scientific advisory board, and receives travel support form Merck. He receives grant support from Merck and Hologic. He is a consultant to Ubiome, VaxGen, Agenovir and Antiva Biosciences. Drs C.J. Wang and J. Sparano have nothing to disclose.

[a] Division of Hematology/Oncology, Department of Medicine, Zuckerberg San Francisco General Hospital, 995 Potrero Avenue, Building 80, 4th Floor, San Francisco, CA 94110, USA; [b] Department of Oncology, Montefiore Medical Center, Albert Einstein College of Medicine, 1695 Eastchester Road, Bronx, NY 10461, USA; [c] Division of Infectious Diseases, Department of Medicine, University of California at San Francisco, 513 Parnassus Avenue, Medical Science Room 420E, Box 0654, San Francisco, CA 94143, USA
* Corresponding author.
E-mail address: joel.palefsky@ucsf.edu

Surg Oncol Clin N Am 26 (2017) 17–31
http://dx.doi.org/10.1016/j.soc.2016.07.010

cancer, anal cancer is typically preceded by precursor lesions. In the general population, anal cancer is a relatively uncommon disease, only accounting for about 3% of all cancers of the gastrointestinal tract.[2] However, the incidence of anal cancer is higher in the human immunodeficiency virus (HIV)-infected population, and it is continuing to increase in the United States.[3] About 80% of all anal cancers arise from the anal canal.[4] In this article, we review the epidemiology of HPV-associated precancerous anal lesions and anal cancer in the HIV-infected population, and highlight some treatment-related issues.

ROLE OF HUMAN PAPILLOMAVIRUS INFECTION

HPV is responsible for 100% of cervical cancers and 88% of anal cancers, with the majority caused by HPV16 or HPV18.[5,6] Almost all (98%) anal cancer tumor specimens from men who were not exclusively heterosexual were positive for HPV, with 73% harboring HPV16.[7] Although the majority of anal cancers associated with HPV are caused by type 16, HPV types 6, 11, and 31 account for 1.4% to 4.1%, and HPV18 accounts for 3.4% to 7%.[8,9] HPV is a small, nonenveloped, double-stranded DNA virus with more than 100 different genotypes identified, of which at least 30 HPV genotypes are sexually transmitted and infect the squamous epithelium of the anogenital tract.[10] HPV is highly prevalent in the young and sexually active population because HPV is transmitted through any sexual activity that involves skin-to-skin or skin-to-mucosa contact, including vaginal, anal, and oral sex.[11] Both symptomatic and asymptomatic individuals can transmit HPV to their sexual partners.[12] Based on conservative assumptions and nationally representative data, more than 50% of sexually active women in the United States are estimated to have been infected by 1 or more genital HPV types at some point in their lifetime.[13] Heterosexual HIV-negative adult men have also been shown to have an overall HPV prevalence of approximately 50%.[14] Concordance of HPV infection between sexual partners is variable and ranges from 40% to 60%, which may be affected by length of sexual relationship, frequency of intercourse, condom use, and number of lifetime sexual partners.[15,16] The overall transmission rate from 1 heterosexual partner to the other over a 6-month period is estimated to be 3.7 cases per 100 person-months.[17] In a 12-month period, the probability for men to acquire a new genital HPV infection is estimated to be 0.29 to 0.39, which is similar to previous estimates for women.[18,19]

The transformation of HPV-infected cells to cancer cells is a multistep process.[20] HPV infects basal cells located in the epithelial transformation zone, a region that extends proximally from the squamocolumnar junction within the rectal columnar mucosa distally to the dentate line. In this area, there is active transition from columnar epithelium to squamous epithelium through the process of squamous metaplasia. Upon entry into the anal epithelium, HPV targets actively proliferating basal cells. E6 and E7 oncoproteins act to enhance cellular proliferation, resulting in increased numbers of infected cells and infectious virions.[21] A spectrum of pathologic changes may occur as a result of HPV infection. Currently, it is believed that low-risk HPV types do not cause malignancy owing to weaker binding of their E6 and E7 to their target proteins, differences in promoter positioning and regulation, and pattern of mRNA splicing compared with E6 and E7 from the high-risk HPV types.[22,23]

The terminology for HPV-associated squamous lesions of the lower anogenital tract has a long history marked by various diagnostic terms derived from multiple specialties. The Lower Anogenital Squamous Terminology (LAST) project aimed to create a histopathologic nomenclature system that reflects current knowledge of HPV biology. Current data support the 2-tiered system of low-grade squamous intraepithelial lesions and high-grade squamous intraepithelial lesions (HSIL),[24] which may be further qualified with the appropriate intraepithelial neoplasia terminology for specific location. Therefore, low-grade squamous intraepithelial lesions include condyloma and anal intraepithelial neoplasia 1, and are not considered to be precancerous. In contrast, HSIL includes p16-positive anal intraepithelial neoplasia 2 and 3. HSIL are considered to be the true cancer precursors.[24]

Infection by multiple oncogenic types of HPV has been associated with a greater likelihood of anal HSIL in HIV-negative men who have sex with men (MSM).[25] HIV-infected individuals, regardless of HIV risk factor, have a high prevalence of HPV infection and are at greater risk for anal squamous intraepithelial lesions, despite good virologic suppression of their HIV.[26,27] In cross-sectional studies, anal HPV infection is almost universal among HIV-infected MSM, with reported prevalence estimates between 87% and 98%.[28–30] A prospective cohort study to assess the natural history of anal HPV infection in HIV-infected MSM in the highly active antiretroviral therapy (HAART) era showed that the incidence of any anal HPV infection and oncogenic anal HPV infection was 21.3 per 100 person-years and 13.3 per 100 person-years, respectively.[31] Twenty percent of these men with an incident HPV infection also had more than 1 new HPV type detected during follow-up.[31] Low CD4 counts are a risk factor for HIV-positive individuals developing anal squamous intraepithelial lesion. Palefsky and colleagues[32] showed that, for HIV-positive men, having CD4 cell counts of less than $200/mm^3$ was associated with a greater than 3-fold increased incidence of progression (based on cytology and/or biopsy) of normal or atypical epithelium to anal squamous intraepithelial lesions, or from anal low-grade squamous intraepithelial lesions to a higher grade lesion.

THE ROLE OF HUMAN IMMUNODEFICIENCY VIRUS AND AIDS

It is estimated that there were approximately 37 million people worldwide living with HIV/AIDS at the end of 2014,[33] including about 1.2 million HIV-infected individuals in the United States.[34] Approximately 1% of women and 28% of men with anal cancer also have HIV infection.[35] Cancer is estimated to be responsible for more than one-third of all deaths in HIV-infected individuals.[36] The immunosuppression associated with HIV infection reduces the ability to control oncogenic viral processes, which could explain the greater risk of infection-related cancer. This hypothesis is supported by a metaanalysis by Grulich and colleagues[37] who compared cancer incidences in population-based cohort studies of persons with HIV infection and organ transplant recipients.

Before the availability of HAART, the estimated incidence of anal cancer among HIV-infected MSM was nearly 60-fold greater than in men in the general population.[38] Since the advent of HAART, the incidence of malignancies associated with Epstein–Barr virus and Kaposi sarcoma herpesvirus has decreased in HIV-infected MSM. However, the incidence of HPV-associated anal cancer has increased (**Fig. 1**). A recent report from the French 2010 survey of deaths in 82,000 HIV-infected patients evaluated the underlying causes of more than 700 deaths from 2000 to 2010. Non–AIDS-defining cancers were the cause of death in 26% of the patients in the most recent period, doubling from 2000. Of the 193 non–AIDS-defining cancers deaths, the commonest were bronchopulmonary malignancies (32%), hepatocellular carcinoma (17%), head and neck cancers (8%), and anal cancer (8%).[39] In a study of 34,189 HIV-infected individuals and 114,260 HIV-uninfected individuals from 13 North American cohorts with follow-up between 1996 and 2007, the unadjusted anal cancer incidence rates per 100,000 person-years were 30 for HIV-infected women,

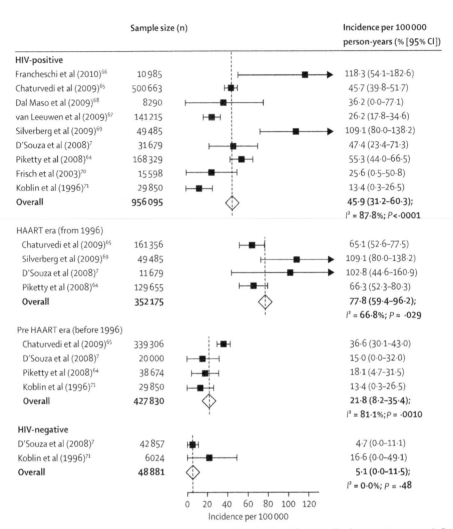

Fig. 1. Incidence of anal cancer in men who have sex with men, by human immunodeficiency virus (HIV) status. The incidence of anal cancer was greater in HIV-positive men than it was in HIV-negative men. In HIV-positive men, the incidence of anal cancer was higher from 1996 onwards (after the introduction of highly active antiretroviral therapy) than it was before 1996. (*From* Machalek DA, Poynten M, Jin F, et al. Anal human papillomavirus infection and associated neoplastic lesions in men who have sex with men: a systematic review and meta-analysis. Lancet Oncol 2012;13(5):495; with permission.)

0 for HIV-uninfected women, 131 per 100,000 for HIV-infected MSM, 46 per 100,000 for other HIV-infected men, and 2 per 100,000 for HIV-uninfected men. Therefore, the incidence of anal cancer in HIV-infected MSM is now estimated to be 80 times higher than men in the general population.[40] This increase in the incidence of anal cancer has been shown to be associated with the HIV epidemic in men.[35]

Immunosuppression plays a pivotal role in the pathogenesis of anal cancer. In a large French HIV cohort study, the risk of anal cancer increased with the time during which the CD4 count was less than 200 cells/mm^3 and viral load was greater than

100,000 copies/mL.[41] A recent analysis from the HIV/AIDS Cancer Match Study, a linkage of population-based state HIV and cancer registries, showed that anal cancer is the third most common cancer occurring in excess in the HIV-positive population. Eighty-three percent of excess cases of anal cancer occurred among MSM, and 71% among those living 5 or more years since AIDS onset.[42]

In the general population, the risk of most cancers increases with age, including cancers frequently diagnosed in HIV-infected individuals.[43] Because effective antiretroviral treatment has greatly prolonged life expectancy, the proportion of the HIV population in older age groups has increased and will likely continue increasing in the future. Yanik and colleagues[44] used a linkage between data from cancer registries in the Surveillance, Epidemiology, and End Results (SEER) program of the National Cancer Institute and Medicare claims (SEER–Medicare)[45] to estimate absolute cancer risk among people age 65 years or older with an HIV diagnosis and evaluate the association between HIV and cancer in this age group. HIV was found to be associated with elevated incidence of anal cancer (adjusted hazard ratio, 34.2) among those aged 65 or older.[44] This highlights a clear need for cancer prevention in this age group and the importance of screening.

TREATMENT OUTCOMES OF HUMAN IMMUNODEFICIENCY VIRUS–POSITIVE ANAL CANCERS

In the general population, concurrent chemoradiotherapy (CRT) with 5-fluorouracil (5-FU) infusion and mitomycin (or cisplatin) has been established as the standard-of-care regimen for nonmetastatic anal cancer.[46–51] Intensity-modulated radiotherapy has also been shown to reduce acute toxicities compared with conventional 3-dimensional radiotherapy.[52,53] For information on treatment of anal cancer in HIV-negative patients (see Rob Glynne-Jones and Sheela Rao's article, "Treatment of the Primary Tumor in Anal Canal Cancers," in this issue).

Outcomes for HIV-infected patients with anal cancer are not as well-described as for HIV-negative individuals. Patients with HIV infection had been excluded from the 3 large randomized phase III trials on anal cancer (ACT I [United Kingdom Co-ordinating Committee on Cancer Research Anal Cancer Trial], RTOG 98–11 [A Phase III Randomized Study of 5-Fluorouracil, Mitomycin, and Radiotherapy Versus 5-Fluorouracil, Cisplatin and Radiotherapy in Carcinoma of the Anal Canal], and ACCORD 03 [A phase III study to evaluate the benefit of cisplatin-fluorouracil–based induction chemotherapy and that of a higher dose of radiotherapy on cancer-free survival]) because of the uncertainties regarding toxicity, compliance, and clinical outcome. When CRT was first applied to HIV-infected patients in the pre-HAART era, reduced doses of radiotherapy and/or chemotherapy were administered as a precaution against the compromised immunologic status and the presumed increased hematologic and mucosal toxicity.[54,55] However, when therapy was applied in standard doses, increased toxicity, requiring treatment breaks or dose reductions, and poorer clinical outcome were reported.[56,57] In 5 studies that included 53 patients, the incidence of grade 3 to 4 skin toxicity was 50% to 78%.[54,56–59] A pretreatment CD4 count of less than 200 was identified as a factor associated with poorer anal cancer control and increased treatment morbidity in a small retrospective cohort.[58]

In the HAART era, reports on clinical outcomes of HIV-infected patients with anal cancer have been conflicting. Immune restoration with effective suppression of HIV viral load and elevation in CD4 count could be achieved in most HIV-infected patients, with a positive impact on treatment-related side effects and compliance. Recent studies with most HIV-infected patients receiving concomitant effective

HAART and CRT found no statistically significant correlation between toxicity and CD4 cell count. Blazy and colleagues[60] reported that high-dose CRT with radiotherapy doses of 60 to 70 Gy with concurrent 5-FU and cisplatin is feasible. Some studies show that HIV-infected patients had comparable disease control and survival to HIV-negative patients,[61–65] whereas others suggested that HIV-positive patients may do worse in terms of enhanced treatment-related toxicity and/or an increased risk for local relapse.[66–70] There are no clear explanations for the differences, or lack of differences, in the outcomes of anal cancer in the HIV-infected versus the HIV-negative population. Almost all of these reports are limited by small patient numbers and the retrospective nature of the data. Wexler and colleagues[65] reported the local failure rate was only 16% in their cohort, but 44% of patients had T1N0 disease, which could reflect the fact that many of the referring providers are experienced in caring for HIV-infected individuals and more likely to examine patients for HSIL and anal cancer. In contrast, one of the largest series of anal cancer patients (total = 107, HIV-infected, HIV-negative) showed that HIV-infected patients had significantly worse overall survival and colostomy free-survival compared with a similar cohort of HIV-negative patients, despite having similar treatment approach, patient adherence, and cancer stage.[70] There were also no differences in radiation-related acute toxicity based on HIV status.

The HPV-associated E5 protein amplifies the mitogenic signals mediated by the epidermal growth factor receptor,[71] which is broadly expressed in epithelial cancers, including squamous cell carcinoma of the anogenital tract and oropharynx.[72,73] There is rationale, therefore, for therapeutically exploiting the association between HPV infection and anal cancer. Cetuximab is a chimeric IgG1 monoclonal antibody that binds epidermal growth factor receptor with high specificity and with greater affinity than its ligands, thus blocking ligand-induced activation of epidermal growth factor receptor.[74] Cetuximab prolongs survival when used in combination with radiation therapy in patients with locally advanced squamous cell carcinoma of the oropharynx,[75,76] another cancer that is typically associated with HPV infection[77–79] but not other head and neck cancers not associated with HPV.[80] Cetuximab also enhances the effectiveness of cisplatin in advanced head and neck carcinoma.[81] Based on these observations, investigators from the AIDS Malignancy Consortium and Eastern Cooperative Oncology Group designed 2 trials that were concurrently conducted to determine the effectiveness of cetuximab plus CRT in patients with HIV infection (AMC045) and without HIV infection (E3205).[82] CRT included cisplatin (75 mg/m^2) and 5-FU (1000 mg/m^2/d × 5 days) × 2 cycles plus radiation therapy (45–54 Gy), plus 2 cycles of neoadjuvant cisplatin/5-FU in the first 28 patients in E3205 before a study amendment. Cetuximab (400 mg/m^2 IV, then 250 mg/m^2 IV weekly × 8 weeks) began 1 week before CRT. When the 2 trials are considered together, a noteworthy finding is that patients with HIV infection had similar clinical outcomes as those who did not have HIV infection, with about 70% being alive and recurrence free at 3 years. Treatment tolerance and the overall side effect profile were also similar in the 2 populations. These findings are consistent with population-based data indicating that, although cancer-specific mortality is increased in HIV-infected subjects compared with the general population for some cancers (eg, colorectal, pancreas, larynx, lung, melanoma, and breast cancer), this is not true for anal cancer.[83] These findings therefore provide additional data indicating that anal cancer in HIV-infected individuals should be treated with curative intent similar to immunocompetent individuals.

Tumor-infiltrating lymphocytes are found in a variety of solid cancers and have been considered to be a manifestation of a host immune response directed against cancer cells. Virus-encoded antigens expressed in the neoplastic cells may represent neoantigens targeted by the immune system. In anal cancer, tumor-infiltrating lymphocytes have been demonstrated to predict overall survival and recurrence-free survival.[84] Some have hypothesized that impaired immune response in HIV-infected patients may allow anal cancer to escape surveillance and results in poorer outcomes. Clearly, the biological basis for poor cancer outcomes in HIV-infected patients requires further study.

MANAGEMENT ISSUES IN HUMAN IMMUNODEFICIENCY VIRUS–POSITIVE PATIENTS

Because HAART allows HIV-infected cohorts to live longer, with a concomitant increased incidence of non–HIV-associated cancers, including anal cancer, concurrent treatment with HAART and anticancer therapy is increasingly common.[85] Extrapolating from treatment studies of HIV-associated lymphomas, concomitant use of HAART and chemotherapy is tolerable in most cases and is not associated with life-threatening toxic effects, similar to those observed in patients with cancer without HIV infection.[86–88] In HIV-infected patients receiving chemotherapy for cancer, most HAART regimens can be safely implemented to suppress viral replication. Typically, the preferred HAART regimens for HIV-infected patients are 2 nucleoside reverse transcriptase inhibitors in combination with a nonnucleoside reverse transcriptase inhibitor, a protease inhibitor (preferably boosted with ritonavir), or an integrase strand transfer inhibitor. Recent guidelines state that integrase strand transfer inhibitor–based regimens may be preferred in cancer patients receiving anticancer treatment because of their favorable drug interaction profile.[89] Zidovudine is often avoided because it commonly causes nausea, anemia, and myelosuppression, which can be potentiated by chemotherapy.[90] Tenofovir may lead to renal dysfunction, particularly in patients receiving other nephrotoxic drugs such as cisplatin. For protease inhibitors and nonnucleoside reverse transcriptase inhibitors, the potential for drug–drug interactions is high because these agents are extensively metabolized by and induce or inhibit the CYP450 system, which mediates the metabolism of more than one-half of all drugs that undergo hepatic metabolism.[91] Protease inhibitors also may act as radiosensitizers by inhibiting proteasome function and causing apoptosis,[92] thereby potentially increasing both tumor control and toxicity.

In HIV-infected patients with cancer, as with other HIV-infected patients, CD4 count, HIV-1 RNA level, and HAART adherence should be monitored.[89] Because CD4 counts can be affected by malignancies or their treatment, CD4 count should be interpreted with caution as an indicator of immunologic response to HAART. For patients with anal cancer who receive pelvic radiation, myelosuppression may be severe since the major source of bone marrow is also radiated. Specifically, the CD4+ T-cell count may fall even more severely and may not readily recover to pretreatment values. In a single institution study of 60 HIV-infected patients with anal cancer, those who received CRT with effective HAART had higher pretreatment CD4 compared those who received CRT without HAART. However, median CD4 at 3 months after anal cancer diagnosis was more than 50% lower than their pretreatment value, and their median CD4 at 12 months after diagnosis was only 200 cells/mm^3.[61] Scatter of radiation may also affect the gut, which is also an important compartment for CD4+ T cells.[93,94] Another group reported that 4 patients (11%) developed opportunistic illnesses such as candida esophagitis during long-term follow-up of their anal cancer.[95] Therefore, antibiotic prophylaxis should be implemented to further reduce infectious complications during the treatment of HIV/AIDS-associated anal cancers based on careful assessment of risk.

The guidelines for prophylaxis against opportunistic infections in patients with HIV take into account risk and history of exposure, as well as the status of the immune system, particularly as reflected by the CD4 count, the receipt of and duration of HAART, and the response to HAART.[96] The guidelines for preventing of infections in patients with cancer are centered on the degree and duration of neutropenia, a key risk factor for infection.[97] CRT also potentiates the neutropenia associated with HIV/AIDS. Granulocyte colony-stimulating factors can reduce the effects of chemotherapy-induced neutropenia, and is often liberally used by oncologists when treating cancer in HIV-infected patients. The caveat is that granulocyte colony-stimulating factors should not be given concurrently with CRT owing to concern for worsening hematologic toxicity.[98] The immunologic deterioration following CRT may have an impact on the clinical course of the HIV disease and may be associated with an increased risk of opportunistic infections and diseases. Both the HIV-related and cancer-related guidelines need to be considered to prevent opportunistic infections in HIV-infected patients with anal cancer.

PREVENTION OF ANAL CANCER IN HUMAN IMMUNODEFICIENCY VIRUS–INFECTED PATIENTS

Anal cancer shares biological similarities with cervical cancer, including detectable precancerous lesions and oncogenic HPV infection. Administration of the prophylactic HPV vaccine before the onset of sexual activity is primary prevention tactic for cervical cancer prevention; this strategy can be mirrored for primary prevention of anal cancer. In 1 double-blind trial, 602 sexually active MSM, age 16 to 26, were randomized to receive 3 doses of the quadrivalent HPV (qHPV) vaccine or placebo and evaluated every 6 months by high-resolution anoscopy (HRA) and HPV testing over 3 years. There was significant reduction of anal HSIL associated with any type of HPV (not only those associated with HPV 6, 11, 16, and 18) in those who received the qHPV compared with those who received the placebo.[99] Wilkin and colleagues[100] evaluated 112 HIV-positive men (ages 27 or older with no evidence of anal HSIL) with the 3-dose course of qHPV vaccine and found that all of these HIV-positive men seroconverted. Therefore, qHPV vaccine has been demonstrated to be both immunogenic and safe in HIV-infected men. The efficacy of primary prevention of anal HSIL in HIV-infected MSM is being evaluated in an ongoing trial.[101]

Deshmukh and colleagues[102] found that qHPV vaccination of HIV-negative MSM age 27 or older treated for anal HSIL reduced the lifetime risk of anal cancer by 60.77% at an incremental increase of cost effectiveness ratios of US$87,240 per quality-adjusted life-year. Their modeling suggests that qHPV vaccination for MSM may decreases their lifetime risk of anal cancer and is a cost-saving strategy because it decreases lifetime costs and increases quality-adjusted life expectancy. In 2015, the 9-valent (9v) HPV vaccine became available. Joura and colleagues[103] evaluated the safety and efficacy of the 9v HPV vaccine through a double-blind international multicenter trial of 14,215 young women randomized to 9v HPV vaccine or qHPV vaccine. The investigators found that the 9v HPV vaccine prevented infection and disease related to HPV 31, 33, 45, 52, and 58 in a susceptible population and generated an antibody response to HPV 6, 11, 16, and 18 that was noninferior to that generated by the qHPV vaccine. From these data, it is assumed that the 9v HPV vaccine will provide the same degree of protection from persistent HPV infections and development of anal HSIL (and possibly progression to anal cancer) in patients without evidence of prior vaccine-type HPV infection.

Similar to cervical cancer screening, secondary prevention of anal cancer consists of detection and treatment of HSIL. Anal HSIL can be detected by anal cytology, digital anorectal examination, HRA, and/or biopsy. Sensitivity of anal cytology is in the range of 50% to 80%, with sensitivity being higher in the HIV-infected population.[104] Individuals with abnormal anal screening cytology are referred for HRA in which the anal canal is examined with a colposcope after the application of 5% acetic acid and/or Lugol's solution and detected lesions are biopsied for histologic diagnosis. Patients with histologic results of anal HSIL are recommended for treatment to prevent progression from anal HSIL to invasive cancer. However, unlike the treatment of cervical HSIL where the entire squamocolumnar junction of the cervix is either ablated or excised, the entire squamocolumnar junction of the anal canal cannot be surgically treated for concerns of stricture or other complications.

Currently, the most commonly used treatment is HRA-directed ablation of apparent anal HSIL lesions. Unfortunately, recurrence rates are very high and frequently additional treatments are needed.[105] The Anal Cancer/HSIL Outcomes Research (ANCHOR) Study is an ongoing phase III, randomized, multiinstitutional trial to determine whether treating anal HSIL is effective in reducing the incidence of anal cancer in HIV-infected men and women.[106] Although definitive efficacy data for an anal cancer screening program are lacking, the potential benefits are significant.[107–109]

SUMMARY

Given the epidemiologic relationship between HIV, HPV, and anal cancer, patients with anal cancer should be screened for HIV infection. Early detection and treatment of anal HPV-related disorders in patients with HIV is a research priority and an unmet need. Clinicians treating HIV-infected patients for anal cancer need to monitor for possible and unexpected interactions between CRT and HIV disease as well as between CRT and HAART. HIV-infected anal cancer patients should be included in clinical trials of both cancer drugs and ART. In the era of HAART, anal cancer can be successfully treated in HIV-positive patients with standard CRT, with clinical outcomes similar to their HIV-negative counterparts. Careful monitoring and management of toxicities are paramount to achieving long-term survival.

REFERENCES

1. Lehtinen M, Dillner J. Clinical trials of human papillomavirus vaccines and beyond. Nat Rev Clin Oncol 2013;10(7):400–10.
2. Siegel RL, Miller KD, Jemal A. Cancer statistics, 2016. CA Cancer J Clin 2016; 66(1):7–30.
3. Patel P, Hanson DL, Sullivan PS, et al. Incidence of types of cancer among HIV-infected persons compared with the general population in the United States, 1992-2003. Ann Intern Med 2008;148(10):728–36.
4. Kauh J, Koshy M, Gunthel C, et al. Management of anal cancer in the HIV-positive population. Oncology (Williston Park) 2005;19(12):1634–8 [discussion: 1638–40, 1645 passim].
5. Arbyn M, de Sanjosé S, Saraiya M, et al. EUROGIN 2011 roadmap on prevention and treatment of HPV-related disease. Int J Cancer 2012;131(9): 1969–82.
6. de Martel C, Ferlay J, Franceschi S, et al. Global burden of cancers attributable to infections in 2008: a review and synthetic analysis. Lancet Oncol 2012;13(6): 607–15.
7. Daling JR, Madeleine MM, Johnson LG, et al. Human papillomavirus, smoking, and sexual practices in the etiology of anal cancer. Cancer 2004;101(2):270–80.

8. Steinau M, Unger ER, Hernandez BY, et al. Human papillomavirus prevalence in invasive anal cancers in the United States before vaccine introduction. J Low Genit Tract Dis 2013;17(4):397–403.

9. Zandberg DP, Bhargava R, Badin S, et al. The role of human papillomavirus in nongenital cancers. CA Cancer J Clin 2013;63(1):57–81.

10. IARC Working Group on the Evaluation of Carcinogenic Risks to Humans. Human papillomaviruses. IARC Monogr Eval Carcinog Risks Hum 2007;90: 1–636.

11. Smyczek P, Singh AE, Romanowski B. Anal intraepithelial neoplasia: review and recommendations for screening and management. Int J STD AIDS 2013;24(11): 843–51.

12. Barr E, Sings HL. Prophylactic HPV vaccines: new interventions for cancer control. Vaccine 2008;26(49):6244–57.

13. Satterwhite CL, Torrone E, Meites E, et al. Sexually transmitted infections among US women and men: prevalence and incidence estimates, 2008. Sex Transm Dis 2013;40(3):187–93.

14. Giuliano AR, Lazcano-Ponce E, Villa LL, et al. The human papillomavirus infection in men study: human papillomavirus prevalence and type distribution among men residing in Brazil, Mexico, and the United States. Cancer Epidemiol Biomarkers Prev 2008;17(8):2036–43.

15. Burchell AN, Tellier PP, Hanley J, et al. Human papillomavirus infections among couples in new sexual relationships. Epidemiology 2010;21(1):31–7.

16. Nyitray AG, Menezes L, Lu B, et al. Genital human papillomavirus (HPV) concordance in heterosexual couples. J Infect Dis 2012;206(2):202–11.

17. Burchell AN, Coutlée F, Tellier PP, et al. Genital transmission of human papillomavirus in recently formed heterosexual couples. J Infect Dis 2011;204(11): 1723–9.

18. Giuliano AR, Lazcano E, Villa LL, et al. Circumcision and sexual behavior: factors independently associated with human papillomavirus detection among men in the HIM study. Int J Cancer 2009;124(6):1251–7.

19. Giuliano AR, Lee JH, Fulp W, et al. Incidence and clearance of genital human papillomavirus infection in men (HIM): a cohort study. Lancet 2011;377(9769): 932–40.

20. Egawa N, Egawa K, Griffin H, et al. Human papillomaviruses; epithelial tropisms, and the development of neoplasia. Viruses 2015;7(7):3863–90.

21. Hamid NA, Brown C, Gaston K. The regulation of cell proliferation by the papillomavirus early proteins. Cell Mol Life Sci 2009;66(10):1700–17.

22. Doorbar J, Quint W, Banks L, et al. The biology and life-cycle of human papillomaviruses. Vaccine 2012;30(Suppl 5):F55–70.

23. Klingelhutz AJ, Roman A. Cellular transformation by human papillomaviruses: lessons learned by comparing high- and low-risk viruses. Virology 2012; 424(2):77–98.

24. Darragh TM, Colgan TJ, Thomas Cox J, et al. The lower anogenital squamous terminology standardization project for HPV-associated lesions: background and consensus recommendations from the College of American Pathologists and the American Society for Colposcopy and Cervical Pathology. Int J Gynecol Pathol 2013;32(1):76–115.

25. Chin-Hong PV, Vittinghoff E, Cranston RD, et al. Age-related prevalence of anal cancer precursors in homosexual men: the EXPLORE study. J Natl Cancer Inst 2005;97(12):896–905.

26. Piketty C, Darragh TM, Heard I, et al. High prevalence of anal squamous intra-epithelial lesions in HIV-positive men despite the use of highly active antiretroviral therapy. Sex Transm Dis 2004;31(2):96–9.
27. Wilkin TJ, Palmer S, Brudney KF, et al. Anal intraepithelial neoplasia in heterosexual and homosexual HIV-positive men with access to antiretroviral therapy. J Infect Dis 2004;190(9):1685–91.
28. Darwich L, Cañadas MP, Videla S, et al. Prevalence, clearance, and incidence of human papillomavirus type-specific infection at the anal and penile site of HIV-infected men. Sex Transm Dis 2013;40(8):611–8.
29. de Pokomandy A, Rouleau D, Ghattas G, et al. Prevalence, clearance, and incidence of anal human papillomavirus infection in HIV-infected men: the HIPVIRG cohort study. J Infect Dis 2009;199(7):965–73.
30. Vajdic CM, van Leeuwen MT, Jin F, et al. Anal human papillomavirus genotype diversity and co-infection in a community-based sample of homosexual men. Sex Transm Infect 2009;85(5):330–5.
31. Hernandez AL, Efird JT, Holly EA, et al. Incidence of and risk factors for type-specific anal human papillomavirus infection among HIV-positive MSM. AIDS 2014;28(9):1341–9.
32. Palefsky JM, Holly EA, Hogeboom CJ, et al. Virologic, immunologic, and clinical parameters in the incidence and progression of anal squamous intraepithelial lesions in HIV-positive and HIV-negative homosexual men. J Acquir Immune Defic Syndr Hum Retrovirol 1998;17(4):314–9.
33. UNAIDS, Fact sheet. 2015. Available at: http://www.unaids.org/en/resources/campaigns/HowAIDSchangedeverything/factsheet. 2015. Accessed April 1, 2016.
34. Centers for Disease Control and Prevention (CDC). HIV in the United States: at a glance. 2015. Available at: http://www.cdc.gov/hiv/statistics/overview/ataglance.html. Accessed April 1, 2016.
35. Shiels MS, Pfeiffer RM, Chaturvedi AK, et al. Impact of the HIV epidemic on the incidence rates of anal cancer in the United States. J Natl Cancer Inst 2012;104(20):1591–8.
36. Bonnet F, Burty C, Lewden C, et al. Changes in cancer mortality among HIV-infected patients: the Mortalite 2005 Survey. Clin Infect Dis 2009;48(5):633–9.
37. Grulich AE, van Leeuwen MT, Falster MO, et al. Incidence of cancers in people with HIV/AIDS compared with immunosuppressed transplant recipients: a meta-analysis. Lancet 2007;370(9581):59–67.
38. Frisch M, Biggar RJ, Goedert JJ. Human papillomavirus-associated cancers in patients with human immunodeficiency virus infection and acquired immunodeficiency syndrome. J Natl Cancer Inst 2000;92(18):1500–10.
39. Morlat P, Roussillon C, Henard S, et al. Causes of death among HIV-infected patients in France in 2010 (national survey): trends since 2000. AIDS 2014;28(8):1181–91.
40. Silverberg MJ, Lau B, Justice AC, et al. Risk of anal cancer in HIV-infected and HIV-uninfected individuals in North America. Clin Infect Dis 2012;54(7):1026–34.
41. Guiguet M, Boué F, Cadranel J, et al. Effect of immunodeficiency, HIV viral load, and antiretroviral therapy on the risk of individual malignancies (FHDH-ANRS CO4): a prospective cohort study. Lancet Oncol 2009;10(12):1152–9.
42. Robbins HA, Pfeiffer RM, Shiels MS, et al. Excess cancers among HIV-infected people in the United States. J Natl Cancer Inst 2015;107(4):dju503.
43. Howlader N, Noone AM, Krapcho M, et al. SEER Cancer statistics review, 1975-2012. Based on November 2014 SEER data submission. Bethesda (MD): National Cancer Institute.

44. Yanik EL, Katki HA, Engels EA. Cancer risk among the HIV-infected elderly in the United States. AIDS 2016;30:1663–8.
45. Engels EA, Pfeiffer RM, Ricker W, et al. Use of Surveillance, Epidemiology, and End Results–Medicare data to conduct case-control studies of cancer among the US elderly. Am J Epidemiol 2011;174(7):860–70.
46. Epidermoid anal cancer: results from the UKCCCR randomised trial of radiotherapy alone versus radiotherapy, 5-fluorouracil, and mitomycin. UKCCCR Anal Cancer Trial Working Party. UK Co-ordinating Committee on Cancer Research. Lancet 1996;348(9034):1049–54.
47. Ajani JA, Winter KA, Gunderson LL, et al. Fluorouracil, mitomycin, and radiotherapy vs fluorouracil, cisplatin, and radiotherapy for carcinoma of the anal canal: a randomized controlled trial. JAMA 2008;299(16):1914–21.
48. Flam M, John M, Pajak TF, et al. Role of mitomycin in combination with fluorouracil and radiotherapy, and of salvage chemoradiation in the definitive nonsurgical treatment of epidermoid carcinoma of the anal canal: results of a phase III randomized intergroup study. J Clin Oncol 1996;14(9):2527–39.
49. Gunderson LL, Winter KA, Ajani JA, et al. Long-term update of US GI intergroup RTOG 98-11 phase III trial for anal carcinoma: survival, relapse, and colostomy failure with concurrent chemoradiation involving fluorouracil/mitomycin versus fluorouracil/cisplatin. J Clin Oncol 2012;30(35):4344–51.
50. James RD, Glynne-Jones R, Meadows HM, et al. Mitomycin or cisplatin chemoradiation with or without maintenance chemotherapy for treatment of squamous-cell carcinoma of the anus (ACT II): a randomised, phase 3, open-label, 2 x 2 factorial trial. Lancet Oncol 2013;14(6):516–24.
51. Northover J, Glynne-Jones R, Sebag-Montefiore D, et al. Chemoradiation for the treatment of epidermoid anal cancer: 13-year follow-up of the first randomised UKCCCR Anal Cancer Trial (ACT I). Br J Cancer 2010;102(7):1123–8.
52. Chuong MD, Freilich JM, Hoffe SE, et al. Intensity-modulated radiation therapy vs. 3D conformal radiation therapy for squamous cell carcinoma of the anal canal. Gastrointest Cancer Res 2013;6(2):39–45.
53. Kachnic LA, Winter K, Myerson RJ, et al. RTOG 0529: a phase 2 evaluation of dose-painted intensity modulated radiation therapy in combination with 5-fluorouracil and mitomycin-C for the reduction of acute morbidity in carcinoma of the anal canal. Int J Radiat Oncol Biol Phys 2013;86(1):27–33.
54. Chadha M, Rosenblatt EA, Malamud S, et al. Squamous-cell carcinoma of the anus in HIV-positive patients. Dis Colon Rectum 1994;37(9):861–5.
55. Peddada AV, Smith DE, Rao AR, et al. Chemotherapy and low-dose radiotherapy in the treatment of HIV-infected patients with carcinoma of the anal canal. Int J Radiat Oncol Biol Phys 1997;37(5):1101–5.
56. Kim JH, Sarani B, Orkin BA, et al. HIV-positive patients with anal carcinoma have poorer treatment tolerance and outcome than HIV-negative patients. Dis Colon Rectum 2001;44(10):1496–502.
57. Place RJ, Gregorcyk SG, Huber PJ, et al. Outcome analysis of HIV-positive patients with anal squamous cell carcinoma. Dis Colon Rectum 2001;44(4):506–12.
58. Hoffman R, Welton ML, Klencke B, et al. The significance of pretreatment CD4 count on the outcome and treatment tolerance of HIV-positive patients with anal cancer. Int J Radiat Oncol Biol Phys 1999;44(1):127–31.
59. Holland JM, Swift PS. Tolerance of patients with human immunodeficiency virus and anal carcinoma to treatment with combined chemotherapy and radiation therapy. Radiology 1994;193(1):251–4.

60. Blazy A, Hennequin C, Gornet JM, et al. Anal carcinomas in HIV-positive patients: high-dose chemoradiotherapy is feasible in the era of highly active antiretroviral therapy. Dis Colon Rectum 2005;48(6):1176–81.
61. Alfa-Wali M, Allen-Mersh T, Antoniou A, et al. Chemoradiotherapy for anal cancer in HIV patients causes prolonged CD4 cell count suppression. Ann Oncol 2012;23(1):141–7.
62. Chiao EY, Giordano TP, Richardson P, et al. Human immunodeficiency virus-associated squamous cell cancer of the anus: epidemiology and outcomes in the highly active antiretroviral therapy era. J Clin Oncol 2008;26(3):474–9.
63. Fraunholz I, Rabeneck D, Gerstein J, et al. Concurrent chemoradiotherapy with 5-fluorouracil and mitomycin C for anal carcinoma: are there differences between HIV-positive and HIV-negative patients in the era of highly active antiretroviral therapy? Radiother Oncol 2011;98(1):99–104.
64. Seo Y, Kinsella MT, Reynolds HL, et al. Outcomes of chemoradiotherapy with 5-Fluorouracil and mitomycin C for anal cancer in immunocompetent versus immunodeficient patients. Int J Radiat Oncol Biol Phys 2009;75(1):143–9.
65. Wexler A, Berson AM, Goldstone SE, et al. Invasive anal squamous-cell carcinoma in the HIV-positive patient: outcome in the era of highly active antiretroviral therapy. Dis Colon Rectum 2008;51(1):73–81.
66. Hogg ME, Popowich DA, Wang EC, et al. HIV and anal cancer outcomes: a single institution's experience. Dis Colon Rectum 2009;52(5):891–7.
67. Munoz-Bongrand N, Poghosyan T, Zohar S, et al. Anal carcinoma in HIV-infected patients in the era of antiretroviral therapy: a comparative study. Dis Colon Rectum 2011;54(6):729–35.
68. Oehler-Janne C, Huguet F, Provencher S, et al. HIV-specific differences in outcome of squamous cell carcinoma of the anal canal: a multicentric cohort study of HIV-positive patients receiving highly active antiretroviral therapy. J Clin Oncol 2008;26(15):2550–7.
69. Meyer JE, Panico VJ, Marconato HM, et al. HIV positivity but not HPV/p16 status is associated with higher recurrence rate in anal cancer. J Gastrointest Cancer 2013;44(4):450–5.
70. Grew D, Bitterman D, Leichman CG, et al. HIV infection is associated with poor outcomes for patients with anal cancer in the highly active antiretroviral therapy era. Dis Colon Rectum 2015;58(12):1130–6.
71. Tsai TC, Chen SL. The biochemical and biological functions of human papillomavirus type 16 E5 protein. Arch Virol 2003;148(8):1445–53.
72. Le LH, Chetty R, Moore MJ. Epidermal growth factor receptor expression in anal canal carcinoma. Am J Clin Pathol 2005;124(1):20–3.
73. Paliga A, Onerheim R, Gologan A, et al. EGFR and K-ras gene mutation status in squamous cell anal carcinoma: a role for concurrent radiation and EGFR inhibitors? Br J Cancer 2012;107(11):1864–8.
74. Blick SK, Scott LJ. Cetuximab: a review of its use in squamous cell carcinoma of the head and neck and metastatic colorectal cancer. Drugs 2007;67(17):2585–607.
75. Bonner JA, Harari PM, Giralt J, et al. Radiotherapy plus cetuximab for squamous-cell carcinoma of the head and neck. N Engl J Med 2006;354(6):567–78.
76. Bonner JA, Harari PM, Giralt J, et al. Radiotherapy plus cetuximab for locoregionally advanced head and neck cancer: 5-year survival data from a phase 3 randomised trial, and relation between cetuximab-induced rash and survival. Lancet Oncol 2010;11(1):21–8.

77. Mork J, Lie AK, Glattre E, et al. Human papillomavirus infection as a risk factor for squamous-cell carcinoma of the head and neck. N Engl J Med 2001;344(15): 1125–31.
78. Herrero R, Castellsagué X, Pawlita M, et al. Human papillomavirus and oral cancer: the International Agency for Research on Cancer multicenter study. J Natl Cancer Inst 2003;95(23):1772–83.
79. D'Souza G, Kreimer AR, Viscidi R, et al. Case-control study of human papillomavirus and oropharyngeal cancer. N Engl J Med 2007;356(19):1944–56.
80. Termine N, Panzarella V, Falaschini S, et al. HPV in oral squamous cell carcinoma vs head and neck squamous cell carcinoma biopsies: a meta-analysis (1988-2007). Ann Oncol 2008;19(10):1681–90.
81. Burtness B, Goldwasser MA, Flood W, et al. Phase III randomized trial of cisplatin plus placebo compared with cisplatin plus cetuximab in metastatic/ recurrent head and neck cancer: an Eastern Cooperative Oncology Group study. J Clin Oncol 2005;23(34):8646–54.
82. Garg M, Lee JY, Kachnic LA, et al. Phase II trials of cetuximab (CX) plus cisplatin (CDDP), 5fluorouracil (5FU) and radiation (RT) in immunocompetent (ECOG 3205) and HIVpositive (AMC045) patients with squamous cell carcinoma of the anal canal (SCAC): safety and preliminary efficacy results. J Clin Oncol 2012;30(Suppl) [abstract: 4030].
83. Coghill AE, Shiels MS, Suneja G, et al. Elevated cancer-specific mortality among HIV-infected patients in the United States. J Clin Oncol 2015;33(21):2376–83.
84. Grabenbauer GG, Lahmer G, Distel L, et al. Tumor-infiltrating cytotoxic T cells but not regulatory T cells predict outcome in anal squamous cell carcinoma. Clin Cancer Res 2006;12(11 Pt 1):3355–60.
85. Rudek MA, Flexner C, Ambinder RF. Use of antineoplastic agents in patients with cancer who have HIV/AIDS. Lancet Oncol 2011;12(9):905–12.
86. Montoto S, Shaw K, Okosun J, et al. HIV status does not influence outcome in patients with classical Hodgkin lymphoma treated with chemotherapy using doxorubicin, bleomycin, vinblastine, and dacarbazine in the highly active antiretroviral therapy era. J Clin Oncol 2012;30(33):4111–6.
87. Ratner L, Lee J, Tang S, et al. Chemotherapy for human immunodeficiency virus-associated non-Hodgkin's lymphoma in combination with highly active antiretroviral therapy. J Clin Oncol 2001;19(8):2171–8.
88. Vaccher E, Spina M, di Gennaro G, et al. Concomitant cyclophosphamide, doxorubicin, vincristine, and prednisone chemotherapy plus highly active antiretroviral therapy in patients with human immunodeficiency virus-related, non-Hodgkin lymphoma. Cancer 2001;91(1):155–63.
89. Gunthard HF, Aberg JA, Eron JJ, et al. Antiretroviral treatment of adult HIV infection: 2014 recommendations of the International Antiviral Society-USA Panel. JAMA 2014;312(4):410–25.
90. Margolis AM, Heverling H, Pham PA, et al. A review of the toxicity of HIV medications. J Med Toxicol 2014;10(1):26–39.
91. Rudek MA, Moore PC, Mitsuyasu RT, et al. A phase 1/pharmacokinetic study of sunitinib in combination with highly active antiretroviral therapy in human immunodeficiency virus-positive patients with cancer: AIDS Malignancy Consortium trial AMC 061. Cancer 2014;120(8):1194–202.
92. Pajonk F, Himmelsbach J, Riess K, et al. The human immunodeficiency virus (HIV)-1 protease inhibitor saquinavir inhibits proteasome function and causes apoptosis and radiosensitization in non-HIV-associated human cancer cells. Cancer Res 2002;62(18):5230–5.

93. Bouma G, Strober W. The immunological and genetic basis of inflammatory bowel disease. Nat Rev Immunol 2003;3(7):521–33.
94. Chun TW, Engel D, Mizell SB, et al. Effect of interleukin-2 on the pool of latently infected, resting CD4+ T cells in HIV-1-infected patients receiving highly active anti-retroviral therapy. Nat Med 1999;5(6):651–5.
95. Fraunholz IB, Haberl A, Klauke S, et al. Long-term effects of chemoradiotherapy for anal cancer in patients with HIV infection: oncological outcomes, immunological status, and the clinical course of the HIV disease. Dis Colon Rectum 2014; 57(4):423–31.
96. Kaplan JE, Benson C, Holmes KK, et al. Guidelines for prevention and treatment of opportunistic infections in HIV-infected adults and adolescents: recommendations from CDC, the National Institutes of Health, and the HIV Medicine Association of the Infectious Diseases Society of America. MMWR Recomm Rep 2009;58(RR-4):1–207 [quiz: CE1–4].
97. Segal BH, Freifeld AG, Baden LR, et al. Prevention and treatment of cancer-related infections. J Natl Compr Canc Netw 2008;6(2):122–74.
98. Bunn PA Jr, Crowley J, Kelly K, et al. Chemoradiotherapy with or without granulocyte-macrophage colony-stimulating factor in the treatment of limited-stage small-cell lung cancer: a prospective phase III randomized study of the Southwest Oncology Group. J Clin Oncol 1995;13(7):1632–41.
99. Palefsky JM, Giuliano AR, Goldstone S, et al. HPV vaccine against anal HPV infection and anal intraepithelial neoplasia. N Engl J Med 2011;365(17): 1576–85.
100. Wilkin T, Lee JY, Lensing SY, et al. Safety and immunogenicity of the quadrivalent human papillomavirus vaccine in HIV-1-infected men. J Infect Dis 2010; 202(8):1246–53.
101. AIDS Malignancy Consortium. Vaccine therapy in preventing human papillomavirus infection in young HIV-positive male patients who have sex with males. In: clinicaltrials.gov. Available at: https://clinicaltrials.gov/ct2/show/NCT01209325. Accessed March 18, 2016.
102. Deshmukh AA, Chhatwal J, Chiao EY, et al. Long-term outcomes of adding HPV vaccine to the anal intraepithelial neoplasia treatment regimen in HIV-positive men who have sex with men. Clin Infect Dis 2015;61(10):1527–35.
103. Joura EA, Giuliano AR, Iversen OE, et al. A 9-valent HPV vaccine against infection and intraepithelial neoplasia in women. N Engl J Med 2015;372(8):711–23.
104. Uronis HE, Bendell JC. Anal cancer: an overview. Oncologist 2007;12(5): 524–34.
105. Stier EA, Chigurupati NL, Fung L. Prophylactic HPV vaccination and anal cancer. Hum Vaccin Immunother 2016;12:1348–51.
106. AIDS Malignancy Consortium. Topical or ablative treatment in preventing anal cancer in patients with HIV and anal high-grade squamous intraepithelial lesions. In: clinicaltrials.gov. Available at: https://clinicaltrials.gov/show/ NCT02135419. Accessed March 18, 2016.
107. Goldstone SE, Johnstone AA, Moshier EL. Long-term outcome of ablation of anal high-grade squamous intraepithelial lesions: recurrence and incidence of cancer. Dis Colon Rectum 2014;57(3):316–23.
108. Park IU, Palefsky JM. Evaluation and management of anal intraepithelial neoplasia in HIV-negative and HIV-positive men who have sex with men. Curr Infect Dis Rep 2010;12(2):126–33.
109. Scholefield JH, Harris D, Radcliffe A. Guidelines for management of anal intraepithelial neoplasia. Colorectal Dis 2011;13(Suppl 1):3–10.

Anal Dysplasia

Craig A. Messick, MD*, Miguel A. Rodriguez-Bigas, MD

KEYWORDS

- Anal dysplasia • HSIL • HGAIN • Anal cytology • High-resolution anoscopy • LSIL
- LGAIN • Squamous cell carcinoma

KEY POINTS

- Recognition of high-grade from low-grade dysplasia is paramount because low-grade dysplasia is not believed to progress to cancer and high-grade dysplastic lesions can be targeted for treatment during high-resolution anoscopy (HRA).
- Treatment strategies vary with multiple options for intra-anal canal and external perianal lesions with high-grade dysplasia all with similar efficacy and recurrence rates.
- HRA is a specialized procedure best suited to identify and treat anal canal and perianal areas with dysplasia; unfortunately, there not enough practitioners using the technique.

Anal dysplasia is a cytopathology term describing specific squamous cell morphology and represents a varying degree of benign changes. Often a source of confusion, the current iteration includes two types, low-grade and high-grade, and carries significant clinical implications. This article updates readers on the current definition of anal dysplasia; describes its incidence and prevalence; defines high-risk populations; and highlights diagnostic, treatment, and long-term management strategies for patients with anal dysplasia.

DEFINITION

In 2001, the Lower Anogenital Squamous Terminology Project, sponsored by the College of American Pathologists and the American Society for Colposcopy and Cervical Pathology, was convened to formalize and uniform a definitive, descriptive definition for anal dysplasia. The group was to formulate a definition using a nomenclature system that would streamline multiple different terms for dysplasia previously derived from a variety of specialties that have accumulated over the preceding century, a source of much confusion among clinicians and specialties. The results were then presented at the Bethesda Consensus Conference to standardize the terminology and ultimately improve diagnostic capability and patient outcomes.[1–3] As a result

The authors have nothing to disclose.
Section of Colon and Rectal Surgery, Surgical Oncology, University of Texas MD Anderson Cancer Center, 1515 Holcombe Blvd, Houston, TX 77030, USA
* Corresponding author.
E-mail address: Cmessick@mdanderson.org

of the conference, anal dysplasia has been simplified into two groups, low-grade and high-grade dysplasia, removing all previously used terminology. Previous terms including anal intraepithelial neoplasia (AIN) I, low-grade dysplasia, mild dysplasia, and condyloma (with appropriate architectural background), are now collectively termed low-grade squamous cell intraepithelial lesions (LSIL), and are not considered precancerous.[1,4] These lesions described by Darragh and colleagues[1] are listed **Table 1**.

The American Society of Colon and Rectal Surgeons recommends using the term low-grade AIN (LGAIN) because the other terms more commonly reflect cytology and not true histologic findings.[5] Terms including Bowen disease, carcinoma in situ, AIN II, AIN III, moderate dysplasia, and high-grade dysplasia are now collectively termed high-grade squamous cell intraepithelial lesions (HSIL) and are considered precursor lesions to cancer, or squamous cell carcinoma (SCC).[4] Likewise, the American Society of Colon and Rectal Surgeons recommend using high-grade AIN (HGAIN) for this group of lesions for the aforementioned reason.[5] As the authors understand current definitions, LSIL and HSIL are used to represent cytology specimens (brushings from the anus) and LGAIN and HGAIN for biopsy or resected tissue specimens.

With the refined consensus definitions, it is anticipated that diagnostic and treating clinicians will have improved accuracy and management outcomes. However, subjective interpretation remains a potential problem with decreased interobserver reproducibility leading to biased specimen diagnoses.[3] Additionally, sampling in the anal canal is challenging because of inherent anatomic constraints. This often results in smaller sample size increasing the likelihood of inadequate tissue for diagnoses, or perhaps even worse, underrepresentation of actual disease.[6]

Table 1
Descriptions of different types of lesions

Name	Description
Low-grade squamous cell intraepithelial lesion (cytology) Low-grade anal intraepithelial neoplasia (tissue)	Proliferation of squamous or metaplastic cells with abnormal nuclear features including increased nuclear size, irregular nuclear membranes, and increased nuclear-to-cytoplasmic ratios. There is little cytoplasmic maturation in the lower third of the epithelium, but maturation begins in the middle third and is relatively normal in the upper third. Mitotic figures are limited to the lower one-third of the epithelium. The presence of diagnostic cytopathic effect of human papilloma virus (koilocytosis) including multinucleation, nuclear enlargement, and pleomorphism accompanied by perinuclear halos without the features of a high-grade lesion.
High-grade squamous cell intraepithelial lesion (cytology) High-grade anal intraepithelial neoplasia (tissue)	Proliferation of squamous or metaplastic squamous cells with abnormal nuclear features including increased nuclear size, irregular nuclear membranes, and increased nuclear-to-cytoplasmic ratio accompanied by mitotic features. There is little or no cytoplasmic differentiation in the middle third and superficial thirds of the epithelium. Mitotic figures are not confined to the lower third of the epithelium and may be found in the middle and/or superficial thirds of the epithelium.

Data from Darragh TM, Colgan TJ, Cox JT, et al. The Lower Anogenital Squamous Terminology Standardization Project for HPV-Associated Lesions: background and consensus recommendations from the College of American Pathologists and the American Society for Colposcopy and Cervical Pathology. J Low Genit Tract Dis 2012;16:205–42.

PREVALENCE OF ANAL DYSPLASIA

For more information on human papilloma virus (HPV) in human immunodeficiency virus (HIV)-positive patients, see Chia-ching J. Wang and colleagues' article, "HIV/AIDS, HPV and Anal Cancer," in this issue. This section focuses on the HIV-negative and immune suppressed, transplanted population and references HIV-positive patients for comparison only. Bowen[7] is credited for the first description of anal dysplasia in a case report in 1912 where it was described as a raised, white scaly lesion. Unfortunately, it was during the era when the cutaneous anal margin skin was not separated from the mucocutaneous anorectal junction in the anal canal, which was later divided because of observed differences in disease behaviors in 1962 by Turell.[8] Despite the initial description more than 100 years ago, significant changes in the terminology and screening efforts have only been established in the last 20 to 30 years, but report a low general prevalence, despite an increase in SCC of the anus by approximately 96% in men and approximately 39% in women over the same period of time.[9,10]

Best reports for the prevalence of anal dysplasia come from within HIV-positive men who have sex with men (MSM), a population practicing anal-receptive intercourse (including AIDS patients), designated a high-risk group. Unfortunately, the percentage of this population varies anywhere from 41% to 97% in HIV-positive men, with less variability in HIV-positive women between 14% and 28%.[11–16] The wide range for anal dysplasia prevalence in the United States likely reflects the variable primary care physician referral strategies for this population to anal dysplasia clinics.[9] These percentages are not expected to change much going forward for the same reason.

The second high-risk population includes HIV-negative, although still immune-suppressed, solid transplant recipients. There have been no formal recommendations for routine anal dysplasia screening for this group, but screening has been suggested because of previous reports. The first report on HPV-related anal dysplasia in transplant recipients was in 1994 by Ogunbiyi and colleagues[17] from the United Kingdom. Their study revealed that 20% of renal transplanted patients had biopsy-proven dysplasia, and of all biopsies (targeted lesions and random if no lesions were seen), 47% were positive for HPV-16, whereas the positivity rate for HPV-16 was 12% in the control arm. Furthermore, they reported that the incidence of anal dysplasia began just after transplant and increased over time up to 10 years where it plateaued at around 30%. With respect to liver transplant patients, Roka and colleagues[18] reported that 24 hours following liver and kidney allograft transplants, anal cytology (formerly termed anal pap smear) revealed HPV DNA in 23% of patients and 15% had high-risk HPV, at that time defined by HPV serotypes 16 and 18. Unfortunately, the patients' HPV status was not known before the transplantations. Although patients undergoing liver transplant had a greater incidence of HPV DNA at 29% compared with renal transplants at 21%, statistical significance was not reached. A more recent study by Grat and colleagues[19] also reported the incidence of HPV infection from anal cytology obtained from 50 liver transplant recipients in the first 3 postoperative weeks. Although they did not report on dysplasia specifically, they reported an HPV infection or detection rate of 18% of liver transplant recipients; 8% had high-risk HPV. More recent reports on the solid organ allograft transplant population are lacking in the literature and should be repeated given new definitions and use of high-resolution anoscopy (HRA) with targeted biopsies.

There are even fewer studies in the general non-high-risk population so the incidence of anal dysplasia and HPV DNA infection is largely unknown; however, relative inferences can be drawn from previous reports. From the study by Ogunbiyi and colleagues,[17] their control arm included 145 normal, healthy, nontransplanted patients and they reported

12% of patients were HPV-16 positive, whereas only 1% of patients had anal dysplasia (AIN II by definition at that time). Perhaps the largest report on the incidence of HGAIN (inferred in the article was caused by HPV-16) was by Johnson and colleagues[10] from the Surveillance, Epidemiology, and End Results database from 1973 to 2000. They reported that during 1973 to 1979, the proportion of anal malignancies classified as being in situ, therefore HGAIN, were similar for men and women at 8.7% and 8.2%, respectively. In the more recent years of the study, however, the percentage of HGAIN was 24.7% for men and 10.4% for women, a dramatic increase and is likely a reflection of the HIV-positive MSM population.[10] The incidence in men (0.09/100,000 in the earlier period) also increased significantly (0.45/100,000 in the more recent period), whereas in women, a more modest increase was seen from 0.12/100,000 in the earlier period to 0.22/100,000 in the more recent period.[10] These data do not include patients with LGAIN or cytology diagnoses LSIL and HSIL. The data must be interpreted carefully, however, because these data do not separate out patients designated high-risk from those who are not considered as such. During their large study period, nearly 30 years, changes in pathologic criteria occurred and need to be considered as a possible contributor to the observed incidence and prevalence increase.

Perhaps the best study to date is the international Human Papilloma Virus Infection in Men study published in 2008 by Giuliano and colleagues.[20] The study enrolled 1160 healthy male subjects with the following eligibility requirements: (1) ages 18 to 70 years; (2) residents of one of three sites (Sao Paulo, Brazil; the state of Morelos, Mexico; or southern Florida, United States); (3) reported no prior diagnosis of penile or anal cancers; (4) have never been diagnosed with genital or anal warts; (5) reported no current symptoms of a sexually transmitted infection or treatment of a sexually transmitted infection; (6) not participating in an HPV vaccine study; (7) no history of HIV or AIDS; (8) no history of imprisonment, homelessness, or drug treatment during the past 6 months; and (9) willing to comply with 10 scheduled visits every 6 months for 4 years with no plans to relocate within the next 4 years. Anal cytology was obtained with swabs and then assessed for HPV DNA using polymerase chain reaction. Cumulatively they reported a prevalence of 65.1% of all males tested HPV-positive with the greatest percentage of HPV-positive men in Brazil (72.3%).[20] Males in the United States had the lowest positive rate at 61.3% followed by Mexico at 61.9%.[20] They reported a large proportion of the HPV-positive patients had multiple HPV serotypes, oncogenic and benign. Their study did not address anal dysplasia; however, it could be inferred from high HPV prevalence in the non-high-risk groups that anal dysplasia may be underappreciated. It is worth noting that the prevalence of LSIL and LGAIN has not been reported outside of the known high-risk patient populations (15%), although their prevalence is expected to be only a small fraction of the patients with anal dysplasia in the general, non-high-risk population. More recently, however, Pineda and colleagues[21] reported a 10-year experience of HRA from their Anal Neoplasia Clinic at the University of California at San Francisco (UCSF). Of the 437 patients who underwent HRA with biopsies and ablative procedures from 1996 to 2006, including 42 patients who were not considered high-risk and were also HIV-negative, 79% had HSIL and 21% had LSIL. The results should be interpreted with caution, however, because their center is a high-volume referral center and the high percentage of non-high-risk patients does not likely reflect the general population.

DIAGNOSTIC TESTS

Diagnostic modalities remain few with the gold standard for diagnosis being tissue biopsy. Digital anorectal examination, where the clinician slowly palpates the lining of the distal rectum and anal canal feeling for subtle surface irregularities, granular or nodular mucosa, and even nodules that may be soft or firm, has been an important screening tool used to palpate lesions inside the anal canal and distal rectum that are not visible with gentle traction. Outside of inflamed hemorrhoids, pathology originating in the anal canal or distal rectum is infrequently discovered using this technique, largely because of their small, flat nature. Small, superficial invasive SCC of the anus may be missed even with significant clinical experience and meticulous digital examination.

Traditional anoscopy has been historically used for visual screening of the anal canal and distal rectum for dysplastic lesions and cancers. Once inserted and the obturator removed, the different anoscopes allow for either on-end visualization or side viewing of the distal rectum, anal transition zone, dentate line, and anal verge. The anoscopes are designed to facilitate biopsy of the lateral walls of the distal rectal vault and anal canal above the dentate line, the insensate internal area within the anal canal. For lesions that either cross or originate at the dentate line, biopsy can be performed; however, infiltration with local analgesic is necessary to avoid significant pain. Despite adequate exposure during traditional anoscopy, most HPV-related dysplasia is not appreciated or detected including HGAIN.[22]

The addition of dilute acetic acid applied via soaked gauze sponges and cotton swabs, a technique adopted from cervical colposcopy, allows lesions within the distal rectum, anal canal, and keratinized skin to become more easily identifiable. Berry and colleagues[23] reported this technique in detail in 2004 and with use of high-magnification microscope or colposcope has been termed a high-resolution anoscopy. On application, areas with high- and low-grade dysplasia display characteristic acetowhite changes and are able to be properly identified under high-magnification. Accurate description of the lesions identified helps differentiate low- from high-grade dysplastic lesions. These lesions may have features of both LGAIN and HGAIN, furthering the point of accurate description being paramount to ensure that the clinician biopsies and potentially treats the precancerous lesions and does not overtreat those lesions that do not require fulguration or additional treatment. These features have been previously described.[24,25] HGAIN lesions more commonly have features including punctuation, pigmentation, dull as opposed to shiny, honey-combing, indistinct borders, large vessels, and lacy metaplasia. LGAIN lesions may also be indistinct, are shiny, and have a mosaic pattern.[24,25] When examining lesions proximal to the dentate line (nonkeratinzed anal canal), application of Lugol solution with a cotton swab better delineates the lesion's borders. When Lugol solution is applied to acetowhite lesions, nonuptake, represented by a light color stain, indicates high-grade dysplasia is present. Darker brown, or mahogany coloration indicates the presence of glycogen and a low-grade dysplastic lesion (**Table 2**).[4]

When HRA is performed routinely in the clinic, detection of anal dysplasia using HRA becomes practical and straightforward. Unfortunately, there are not enough practitioners performing HRA and until more arise anal cytology may be considered and acceptable alternative. This simple test should be relatively painless and requires a minimal amount of time to perform appropriately. A Dacron swab (not cotton) is gently placed into the anal canal until impedance is reached (usually 4–5 cm). It is critical to perform this before use of any lubricant because of interference with the test. The Dacron swab is twirled while moved in a circular fashion within the anal canal. This is performed from the deepest point of entry all the way out of the anal verge. Twenty to 30 seconds should be allotted for this procedure to ensure the adequacy of the sample. The swab should be swished into the collection fluid for another 20 to 30 seconds and the tip cut off and sent in the specimen container. Using this technique, the

Table 2
Features of HGAIN and LGAIN lesions

High-Resolution Anoscopy Lesion Descriptions	With Use of 5% Acetic Acid	With Application of Lugol Solution
High-grade anal intraepithelial neoplastic lesions	Flat or slightly raised (thickened epithelium); acetowhite lesions with dull, not shiny appearance; presence of abnormal vascularity displaying coarse punctuation (on-end vessels); mosaic pattern; and honey-combing	Lugol-negative (no uptake leaving a light brown color)
Low-grade anal intraepithelial neoplastic lesions	Flat, or raised epithelium, mildly acetowhite, shiny in appearance, and may have lacy appearance (lacy metaplasia), fine punctuation and scalloping	Lugol-positive (uptake leaving a mahogany, dark brown color)

sensitivity to detect HSIL in the anal canal is between 50% and 80%[22,26] and is similar when compared with cervical cytology performing traditional Pap smears. The varied sensitivity is likely caused by the higher prevalence of disease in high-risk, HIV-positive MSM compared with non-high-risk HIV-negative non-MSM and women.

TREATMENT OF ANAL DYSPLASIA

There are several treatment options for patients with anal dysplasia. Because LSIL and LGAIN lesions have been deemed nonprecursors to cancer, their treatment is decided on by the clinician's individual preference; however, it does not likely need to be treated at all from the current understanding of disease progression. The remainder of this section focuses on treatment of HSIL and HGAIN. The data published on treatment largely comes from the high-risk populations as previously defined. There are limited data on the non-high-risk patients with HSIL and HGAIN, but some data have been published to date from the high-risk centers.

Regardless of treatment choice, the ultimate goal is to prevent anal SCC formation from known high-risk lesions. A secondary goal is to clear all high-grade dysplasia to normal tissue and minimize disease recurrence without causing defecatory dysfunction. Unfortunately, high-grade dysplasia is well documented to recur. Goldstone and colleagues[27] reported a comprehensive review of their high-risk patient population in HIV-positive and -negative MSM in 2014. At a median of 2.2 years, out of 456 HIV-positive and 271 HIV-negative MSM, they reported the median time to HSIL/HGAIN recurrence was 6.8 and 6.9 months, respectively. These authors also reported that within the first year of an HRA following ablation, 53% (95% confidence interval, 49%–58%) and 49% (95% confidence interval, 43%–55%) of HIV-positive and HIV-negative patients had recurred, respectively.[27] This rate increased to 77% in HIV-positive and 66% HIV-negative MSM by year 3 indicating that even after a several year period, patients are still at risk for recurrence. In this study, five HIV-positive MSM progressed to invasive anal SCC at 3 years (1.97%; 95% confidence interval, 0.73%–5.2%).[27] Johnstone and colleagues[24] reported similar data in 2015 for perianal lesions, those on the anal verge and margin. Although there are data on the use of CO_2 laser ablation as a fulguration technique, the cumulative experience has not shown laser to be a superior therapy and as such, the authors use electrocautery for ablation. There is essentially no data on dysplasia recurrence and natural history in patients who are not considered high-risk. The only report to date is from the UCSF group who reported on 42 patients (30 male) with a mean age of 39 years. These patients were all HIV-negative and not practicing anal-receptive intercourse. A total of 33 of 42 patients had HSIL. Over a 10-year period, there were recurrences in 45% of patients with HSIL, whereas no patient with LSIL recurred. One patient with LSIL developed HSIL and another patient with HSIL progressed to invasive SCC anus (2.4%).[21] The longer natural history has yet to be described in those patients not considered high-risk.

Treatment is considered as targeted for anal canal, anal verge, and margin. When there is HSIL/HGAIN outside the anal canal on the anal verge or margin, there usually is disease inside the anal canal and one should be aggressive in localizing the HGAIN lesion. Alternatively, if HISL/HGAIN is found inside the anal canal, it may not necessarily be on the perianal skin. The authors take a conservative approach for disease on the keratinized portion of the anal canal, verge, and margin because of scar formation from fibrosis. Given the likelihood of repeated treatments to remove or destroy HGAIN, frequent, repeated thermal ablation can result in significant scaring and possible anal stricture. However, because of the rapid cellular turnover in the anal canal in the mucosalized portion proximal to the dentate line, scaring is not as much a concern and repeated ablation or resections from biopsy is often performed. This area happens to be the location at greatest risk for HPV-related changes.

For external HGAIN, in immune-competent patients, topical application of imiquimod (Aldara), a cytokine stimulator, has shown good success at eradication of dysplasia. Topical 5-fluorouracil (Efudex), an antimetabolite that interferes with the synthesis of DNA and to a lesser extent inhibits RNA formation, has also been used in the treatment of HGAIN. There are no studies to date in the non-high-risk population that address any treatment efficacy, outcomes, and recurrence risk. In 2014, Richel and colleagues[28] published a randomized, open-label control trial comparing topical imiquimod (54 patients), 5-fluorouracil (48 patients), and electrocautery (46 patients) in the high-risk groups. Interestingly, for lesions that were considered external (perianal), imiquimod was successful at achieving complete response in 100% of patients compared with 57% treated with fluorouracil, and 75% with electrocautery. Overall, considering all sites of HGAIN, complete response was seen in 24%, 17%, and 39% of lesions, respectively. By week 72, however, recurrent HGAIN was seen in 71% of patients treated with imiquimod, 58% of patients treated with fluorouracil, and 68% of patients treated with electrocautery. The use of imiquimod requires a competent immune system and in patients with AIDS, expectations should be less because it is a cytokine modulator and essentially interferes with cellular signaling directed from the virus.[29,30] Topical 5-fluorouracil does not require a competent immune system and may have better results in patients with AIDS.[31]

Other alternative treatments include trichloroacetic acid (TCA) at varying concentrations between 35% and 80%, infrared coagulation (IRC), and photodynamic therapy (PDT). These alternative forms of topical therapy have had differing effects on the treatment of anal dysplasia and are unfortunately fraught with similar recurrence rates. In 2014, Cranston and colleagues[32] reported promising results in 98 HSILs from 72 patients treated only with in-office TCA (concentration not noted) by two certified HRA physicians. Of the 98 lesions identified, 77 (78.6%) resolved to normal epithelium or had developed LSIL/LGAIN on HRA during routine 3 to 6 month follow-up. Forty-eight (49.0%) and 27 (27.6%) of lesions resolved with one and two TCA treatments, respectively. A single lesion (1%) required four TCA treatments for complete resolution. Twenty patients had 21 lesions that persisted requiring alternative therapy regimens. They reported same-site recurrences in 15.1% of the 53 patients (20.8% recurrences when including new lesions at adjacent sites). Seventeen patients had new lesions diagnosed at new locations altogether.[32] PDT has had some reports dating back to 2004. This method involves oral administration of the photosensitizer delta-aminolevulinic acid followed by PDT treatment to the entire anal canal, verge, and margin approximately 4 hours after ingestion. Most reports are limited to case reports or small series, but Runfola and colleagues[33] reported results in five patients (two with Bowen disease) and complete resolution of disease with one of two patients developing a recurrence at 4 years posttreatment. Another study reported at least downgrading in the severity of anal dysplasia in all of the 12 patients.[34] A more recent study by Welbourn and colleagues[35] reported resolution of AIN in 6 of 10 patients treated with PDT; however, recurrence was subsequently documented in three of those complete responders in short follow-up. IRC use for anal dysplasia was first reported by Goldstone and colleagues[36] in 2005. It has since been reported several times with varying results. In the original report, 68 patients were included and 165 lesions were treated (mean 1.6 lesions; range 1–5). Following IRC, only 46 (28%) lesions persisted; however, 44 patients (65%) developed a new or persistent HSIL within a median time of 217 days (range, 27–566 days). The remaining 24 patients (35%) were free of HSIL at a median of 413 days (range, 162–1313 days). Second or third time treatment of new or persistent HSIL decreased to 58% and 40%, respectively, yielding a probability of cure at approximately 72%.[36] A follow-up study recently published showed improved outcomes. Sirera and colleagues[37] (part of the HIV-HPV study group) reported resolution of HSIL/HGAIN in 87.5% of patients (49/56), at mean follow-up of 25 (range, 12–60) months. After the 12 months of post-IRC follow-up, only seven patients (12.5% recurrence) had abnormal anal cytology, and recurrent disease (HGAIN) was then biopsy-proven at a mean of 30 (range, 18–43) months.[37]

These data are largely limited to the high-risk patient population and their extrapolation to non-high-risk patients should be considered cautiously. Although it would seem intuitive that the natural history, treatment outcomes, recurrence rates, and progression to anal SCC would be improved in an immune-competent population, the data are absent to support that notion. This is largely caused by an inability to screen a population not identified as at risk. For patients with HSIL/HGAIN who are not high-risk, at least annual follow-up has been suggested given the low likelihood of progression to cancer; however, because no long-term data exist to attest to that, it seems just as reasonable to consider closer surveillance because HSIL/HGAIN has been shown to recur within 6 months following treatment. The authors consider a 3- to 4-month follow-up surveillance program for all patients with HSIL/HGAIN, HIV-positive or negative, transplanted or not, because having a high-grade lesion should consider the patient at greater risk than the general population for development of additional anal dysplasia. Treatment of LSIL/LGAIN is not necessary unless lesions are bulky or causing symptoms to the patient. They are now understood to be very low risk for progressing to high-grade dysplasia or cancer, but should be followed at 6-month intervals with HRA to reassess for potentially missed HSIL/HGAIN, or interval development of new lesions. HRA with targeted ablation for intra-anal canal HGAIN/HSIL lesions should be performed at 3- to 4-month intervals with repeated procedures as recurrent lesions or new lesions are identified. For HSIL/HGAIN lesions noted to be on the skin-bearing portion of the anal canal, verge and margin, target ablation for small lesions or topical treatment is appropriate for 3 months with a repeat HRA to reassess for recurrences or new lesions. A summary of the treatment options with outcomes is listed in **Table 3**.

Table 3
Summary of treatment options for anal neoplasia

Treatment Type	Recurrence Rates	
High-resolution anoscopy with targeted ablation Laser or electrocautery[21,27]	HIV-positive MSM 53% at 1 y, 77% at 3 y HIV-negative MSM 49% at 1 y, 66% at 3 y UCSF Group: non-high-risk patients 45% at 10 y	
Topical creams (perianal verge and margin)[28]	*Primary Response Rate*	*Recurrence Rate*
Imiquimod (Aldara)	100%	71% at 72 wk
5-Fluorouracil (Efudex)	57%	58% at 72 wk
Trichloroacetic acid, 35%–80% concentrations[32]	79% after one application 49% after two applications 28% after three applications	15% same site 21% adjacent site 17% new site
Photodynamic therapy[33,35]	5/5 patients with complete response 6/10 patients with complete response	1/2 patients at 4 y 3/10 patients short follow-up
Infrared coagulation[37]	88% at 25 mo	13% at 30 mo

Abbreviation: non-high risk, heterosexual, nontransplant population.

SUMMARY

Updated definitions have allowed clinicians to more accurately diagnose and treat HPV-related dysplasia in the anal canal and anal margin. Although most published data reflect a high-risk population consisting of HIV-positive/AIDS patients, especially MSM, and solid organ transplant recipients, there are limited studies that offer insight into all other patients who develop anal neoplasia. There are good data from high-risk populations that should serve as a guide for management of non-high-risk patients until studies reflective of the general population are reported. HRA with targeted biopsy and ablation should be considered standard of care at this point for these patients with follow-up every 3 to 4 months for repeat evaluations until the disease is no longer present. Surgical management of this infectious disease should be considered carefully because repeat ablations or resections may be required leading to scaring of the anus and ultimately stenosis or other defecatory dysfunction. Current data do not support the use of one modality over another, but selection of treatment choice should be the modality with which each clinician is most familiar and comfortable.

REFERENCES

1. Darragh TM, Colgan TJ, Cox JT, et al. The Lower Anogenital Squamous Terminology Standardization Project for HPV-Associated Lesions: background and consensus recommendations from the College of American Pathologists and the American Society for Colposcopy and Cervical Pathology. J Low Genit Tract Dis 2012;16(3):205–42.
2. Darragh TM, Colgan TJ, Thomas Cox J, et al. The Lower Anogenital Squamous Terminology Standardization project for HPV-associated lesions: background and consensus recommendations from the College of American Pathologists and the American Society for Colposcopy and Cervical Pathology. Int J Gynecol Pathol 2013;32(1):76–115.

3. Stoler MH, Schiffman M. Interobserver reproducibility of cervical cytologic and histologic interpretations: realistic estimates from the ASCUS-LSIL Triage Study. JAMA 2001;285(11):1500–5.
4. Palefsky J. Human papillomavirus and anal neoplasia. Curr HIV/AIDS Rep 2008; 5(2):78–85.
5. Steele SR, Varma MG, Melton GB, et al. Practice parameters for anal squamous neoplasms. Dis Colon Rectum 2012;55(7):735–49.
6. Stoler MH, Vichnin MD, Ferenczy A, et al. The accuracy of colposcopic biopsy: analyses from the placebo arm of the Gardasil clinical trials. Int J Cancer 2011; 128(6):1354–62.
7. Bowen J. Precancerous dermatoses: a study of two cases of chronic atypical epithelial proliferation. J Cutan Dis Syph 1912;30:241.
8. Turell R. Epidermoid squamous cell cancer of the perianus and anal canal. Surg Clin North Am 1962;42:1235–41.
9. Chiao EY, Krown SE, Stier EA, et al. A population-based analysis of temporal trends in the incidence of squamous anal canal cancer in relation to the HIV epidemic. J Acquir Immune Defic Syndr 2005;40(4):451–5.
10. Johnson LG, Madeleine MM, Newcomer LM, et al. Anal cancer incidence and survival: the surveillance, epidemiology, and end results experience, 1973-2000. Cancer 2004;101(2):281–8.
11. Durante AJ, Williams AB, Da Costa M, et al. Incidence of anal cytological abnormalities in a cohort of human immunodeficiency virus-infected women. Cancer Epidemiol Biomarkers Prev 2003;12(7):638–42.
12. Friedman HB, Saah AJ, Sherman ME, et al. Human papillomavirus, anal squamous intraepithelial lesions, and human immunodeficiency virus in a cohort of gay men. J Infect Dis 1998;178(1):45–52.
13. Goldstone SE, Winkler B, Ufford LJ, et al. High prevalence of anal squamous intraepithelial lesions and squamous-cell carcinoma in men who have sex with men as seen in a surgical practice. Dis Colon Rectum 2001;44(5):690–8.
14. Hillemanns P, Ellerbrock TV, McPhillips S, et al. Prevalence of anal human papillomavirus infection and anal cytologic abnormalities in HIV-seropositive women. AIDS 1996;10(14):1641–7.
15. Melbye M, Smith E, Wohlfahrt J, et al. Anal and cervical abnormality in women: prediction by human papillomavirus tests. Int J Cancer 1996;68(5):559–64.
16. Sayers SJ, McMillan A, McGoogan E. Anal cytological abnormalities in HIV-infected homosexual men. Int J STD AIDS 1998;9(1):37–40.
17. Ogunbiyi OA, Scholefield JH, Raftery AT, et al. Prevalence of anal human papillomavirus infection and intraepithelial neoplasia in renal allograft recipients. Br J Surg 1994;81(3):365–7.
18. Roka S, Rasoul-Rockenschaub S, Roka J, et al. Prevalence of anal HPV infection in solid-organ transplant patients prior to immunosuppression. Transpl Int 2004; 17(7):366–9.
19. Grat M, Grąt K, Hołówko W, et al. Initial prevalence of anal human papilloma virus infection in liver transplant recipients. Transpl Int 2014;27(8):816–23.
20. Giuliano AR, Lazcano-Ponce E, Villa LL, et al. The human papillomavirus infection in men study: human papillomavirus prevalence and type distribution among men residing in Brazil, Mexico, and the United States. Cancer Epidemiol Biomarkers Prev 2008;17(8):2036–43.
21. Pineda CE, Berry JM, Jay N, et al. High resolution anoscopy in the planned staged treatment of anal squamous intraepithelial lesions in HIV-negative patients. J Gastrointest Surg 2007;11(11):1410–5 [discussion: 1415–6].

22. Berry JM, Palefsky JM, Jay N, et al. Performance characteristics of anal cytology and human papillomavirus testing in patients with high-resolution anoscopy-guided biopsy of high-grade anal intraepithelial neoplasia. Dis Colon Rectum 2009;52(2):239–47.

23. Berry JM, Jay N, Palefsky J, et al. State-of-the-art of high-resolution anoscopy as a tool to manage patients at risk for anal cancer. Semin Colon Rectal Surg 2004; 15(4):218–26.

24. Johnstone AA, Silvera R, Goldstone SE. Targeted ablation of perianal high-grade dysplasia in men who have sex with men: an alternative to mapping and wide local excision. Dis Colon Rectum 2015;58(1):45–52.

25. Jay N, Berry JM, Hogeboom CJ. Colposcopic appearance of anal squamous intra-epithelial lesions: relationship to histopathology. Dis Colon Rectum 1997; 40(8):919–28.

26. Cranston RD, Darragh TM, Holly EA, et al. Self-collected versus clinician-collected anal cytology specimens to diagnose anal intraepithelial neoplasia in HIV-positive men. J Acquir Immune Defic Syndr 2004;36(4):915–20.

27. Goldstone SE, Johnstone AA, Moshier EL. Long-term outcome of ablation of anal high-grade squamous intraepithelial lesions: recurrence and incidence of cancer. Dis Colon Rectum 2014;57(3):316–23.

28. Richel O, de Vries HJ, van Noesel CJ, et al. Comparison of imiquimod, topical fluorouracil, and electrocautery for the treatment of anal intraepithelial neoplasia in HIV-positive men who have sex with men: an open-label, randomised controlled trial. Lancet Oncol 2013;14(4):346–53.

29. Baulon E, Vautravers A, Rodriguez B, et al. Imiquimod and immune response modifiers in gynaecology. Gynecol Obstet Fertil 2007;35(2):149–57 [in French].

30. Tyring SK. Immune-response modifiers: a new paradigm in the treatment of human papillomavirus. Curr Ther Res 2000;61(9):584–96.

31. Weis SE. Current treatment options for management of anal intraepithelial neoplasia. Onco Targets Ther 2013;6:651–65.

32. Cranston RD, Baker JR, Liu Y, et al. Topical application of trichloroacetic acid is efficacious for the treatment of internal anal high-grade squamous intraepithelial lesions in HIV-positive men. Sex Transm Dis 2014;41(7):420–6.

33. Runfola MA, Weber TK, Rodriguez-Bigas MA, et al. Photodynamic therapy for residual neoplasms of the perianal skin. Dis Colon Rectum 2000;43(4):499–502.

34. Webber J, Fromm D. Photodynamic therapy for carcinoma in situ of the anus. Arch Surg 2004;139(3):259–61.

35. Welbourn H, Duthie G, Powell J, et al. Can photodynamic therapy be the preferred treatment option for anal intraepithelial neoplasia? Initial results of a pilot study. Photodiagnosis Photodyn Ther 2014;11(1):20–1.

36. Goldstone SE, Kawalek AZ, Huyett JW. Infrared coagulator: a useful tool for treating anal squamous intraepithelial lesions. Dis Colon Rectum 2005;48(5):1042–54.

37. Sirera G, Videla S, Piñol M, et al. Long-term effectiveness of infrared coagulation for the treatment of anal intraepithelial neoplasia grades 2 and 3 in HIV-infected men and women. AIDS 2013;27(6):951–9.

Diagnosis and Diagnostic Imaging of Anal Canal Cancer

Kristen K. Ciombor, MD, MSCI[a],*, Randy D. Ernst, MD[b],
Gina Brown, MBBS, MRCP, FRCR[c]

KEYWORDS

- Anal canal cancer • Magnetic resonance imaging
- 18F-fluorodeoxyglucose positron emission tomography • Anoscopy
- Endoanal ultrasound

KEY POINTS

- Anal canal cancer can present with rectal bleeding, pain, or change in bowel habits and is often a delayed diagnosis owing to the similarity of symptoms to common benign conditions.
- Staging procedures for anal canal cancer can include anoscopy, biopsy, computed tomography, MRI, endoanal ultrasound imaging, and/or 18F-fluorodeoxyglucose-PET.
- Imaging modalities for detection, staging, evaluation of treatment response and surveillance of anal canal cancer are sensitive and robust.

INTRODUCTION

Anal canal cancer is a relatively uncommon malignancy, with an incidence of approximately 30,000 cases annually worldwide.[1] Owing to the unique location and anatomy of this malignancy, careful examination and diagnostic procedures are necessary for optimal staging and treatment. This article focuses on the underlying anatomy of the anorectal region, important imaging characteristics of the anus, common clinical presentations of anal canal cancer, and the diagnostic procedures required for adequate staging and treatment of this cancer type.

Disclosure Statement: G. Brown is supported by the UK NIHR Biomedical Research Centre.
[a] Division of Medical Oncology, Department of Internal Medicine, The Ohio State University, A445A Starling Loving Hall, 320 West 10th Avenue, Columbus, OH 43210, USA; [b] Division of Diagnostic Imaging, Department of Diagnostic Radiology, The University of Texas MD Anderson Cancer Center, Unit 1473, PO Box 301402, Houston, TX 77230-1402, USA; [c] Department of Radiology, The Royal Marsden NHS Foundation Trust and Imperial College London, Downs Road, Sutton, Surrey SM2 5PT, UK
* Corresponding author.
E-mail address: Kristen.ciombor@osumc.edu

ANATOMY OF THE ANUS

The anus drains the last 3 to 5 cm of the gastrointestinal tract through the internal and external anal sphincters, extending from the dentate line to the anal verge and perineum (**Fig. 1**). The anatomic anal canal goes from the dentate line or valves of Morgagni to the anal verge (**Fig. 2**). The surgical anal canal is longer than the anatomic canal and starts at the level of the anorectal ring just above the anal columns of Morgagni and extends to the anal verge or margin.[2] The muscular wall of the rectum, the muscularis propria, is covered with columnar epithelium. This columnar epithelium overlies the upper one-half or two-thirds of the internal sphincter and internal hemorrhoid plexus. The lining changes from columnar to transitional epithelium and at the free edge of the columns of Morgagni to squamous epithelium. The irregular junction indicates the dentate or pectinate line, with biopsy showing islands of squamous epithelium in between columnar epithelium.[2]

The inner circular muscle of the muscularis propria becomes the internal sphincter in the anus and is covered by squamous epithelium. The conjoined longitudinal muscle of the muscularis propria becomes the intersphincteric plane. The external sphincter complex is composed of the most inferior part of the levator ani muscle, the puborectalis sling, and the external sphincter muscles. The upper border of the puborectalis sling forms the upper edge of the surgical anal canal. True squamous skin with sweat glands and hair follicles covers the anal verge.[3,4]

CLINICAL PRESENTATION

Patients diagnosed with anal canal cancer often present with anorectal pain or bleeding, but these symptoms occur in only approximately one-half of patients. Other clinical manifestations of anal canal cancer include anorectal fullness, pruritus, and change in bowel habits.[5,6] More advanced tumors can cause fecal incontinence or weight loss. Many patients with anal cancer come to the attention of physicians with complaints of hemorrhoidal-type bleeding or pain, and about one-half are not diagnosed until more than 24 months after symptom onset.[6] Because the symptoms of anal cancer can mimic those of more common, benign conditions, the diagnosis of anal cancer is often delayed. In some cases, patients are entirely asymptomatic from their anal cancer.

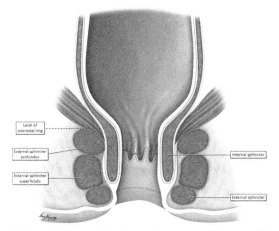

Fig. 1. Anatomy of the anal canal, including relevant musculature. (*Courtesy of* Kelly M. Kage, BS, MFA, University of Texas MD Anderson Cancer Center, Houston, TX.)

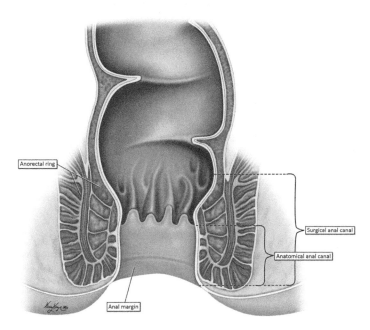

Fig. 2. Anatomy of the anatomic and surgical anal canal. (*Courtesy of* Kelly M. Kage, BS, MFA, University of Texas MD Anderson Cancer Center, Houston, TX.)

Patients being evaluated for anal cancer should have a thorough history of potential risk factors taken, including human immunodeficiency virus (HIV)/AIDS, non–HIV-related immunosuppression, organ transplantation, chronic steroid use, receptive anal intercourse, cigarette smoking, and human papilloma virus infection.[7] In addition to these, a history of cervical, vulvar, or vaginal cancer can be a significant risk factor as well. In high-risk populations, some advocate for anal cancer screening to decrease the incidence of anal cancer,[8] although no formal guidelines currently exist for routine anal cancer screening.

DIAGNOSIS AND PROCEDURES

In patients with worrisome anorectal complaints, a thorough physical examination, including visual inspection of the perirectal area and a digital rectal reexamination, must be undertaken. A digital rectal reexamination can identify the primary lesion, determine whether there is sphincter invasion, and/or fixation of the tumor, and identify perirectal lymphadenopathy, if present.[9] In addition, the presence or absence of inguinal lymphadenopathy must be assessed. After a complete physical examination has been performed, histologic diagnosis of anal cancer is generally determined through biopsies obtained during an examination under anesthesia with anoscopy or proctosigmoidoscopy; this is also often necessary to ensure patient tolerance of a complete examination.[9] Further information about the primary tumor, such as anal cancer size, depth, sphincter involvement, and local lymph node involvement, can be elicited from endoanal ultrasound or MRI, if desired.[10–12]

With respect to MRI, the recent widespread success of this imaging modality for rectal cancer staging could benefit anal cancer staging given the similar tumor location. In primary rectal cancer, high-resolution T2-weighted imaging is the best MRI sequence. The T2 sequence consists of thin section (3 mm) axial images obtained orthogonal to the tumor plane, with an in-plane resolution of 0.5 to 0.8 mm. This technique allows differentiation between rectal tumors confined within the rectal wall (stage T2 tumors) and those that extend beyond the muscularis propria (stage T3 tumors). Most important, the depth of invasion outside the muscularis propria can be assessed with a high degree of accuracy.[13] In addition, high-resolution T2-weighted images allow the morphologic assessment of pelvic nodes, thereby improving accuracy in the characterization of nodes as benign or malignant, because size criteria have proved to be of limited value.[3,14] Furthermore, MRI may be better for localization of suspicious lymph nodes outside of the field of view of endoscopic ultrasound imaging.

Once evaluation of the primary tumor has been completed, computed tomography of the chest, abdomen, and pelvis should be performed to evaluate for lymphadenopathy and distant metastasis. Any clinically enlarged or radiographically abnormal inguinal lymph nodes must be histologically evaluated through biopsy, as this determines staging and potential radiation dosing required. 18F-fluorodeoxyglucose PET/computed tomography can also identify suspicious lymph nodes or distant metastases not detected by physical examination,[15,16] and pretreatment PET/computed tomography maximum standardized uptake value is strongly associated with primary tumor stage and histology.[17] Future hybrid PET-MRI scanners may improve the diagnostic performance of 18F-fluorodeoxyglucose PET.[18]

In addition to imaging, patients with a new diagnosis of anal cancer should undergo basic laboratory studies, including a complete blood count, renal and hepatic function tests, and HIV status, if not already known. Women should also undergo a Papanicolaou test to screen for precancerous and cancerous lesions in the cervix, and men should undergo penile examination to exclude premalignant or malignant lesions there as well.

ANORECTAL ANATOMY AND IMAGING
The Sphincter Complex and Pelvic Floor

The continuity of the muscularis propria and internal sphincter is well depicted on a coronal MRI (**Fig. 3**A). The intersphincteric plane that separates internal sphincter from the somatic muscle "sheet" is contiguous with the external sphincter. The most proximal portion of this sheet is made up of the levator muscles, which are attached at the sacrum, lateral pelvic sidewall, and symphysis pubis to form a hammocklike muscular diaphragm of the pelvic floor. The most distal fibers of the levator blend with the uppermost fibers of the puborectalis muscle (**Fig. 3**B). The latter forms a sling that creates the acute angle of the anorectal junction and is anchored to the inferior public rami. Fibers of the puborectalis sling in turn blend with the external sphincter. The lower fibers of the external sphincter terminate 3 to 4 mm below the internal sphincter at the anal verge.

The Anal Canal

The surface mucosal layer in the anal canal is less than 1 mm in thickness and is seen as a discrete, low signal intensity layer. Below this is the thicker submucosal layer containing lymphatics and vasculature, which is of intermediate signal intensity compared with fluid or muscle and has a thickness of several millimeters. The internal sphincter is a thin, 1- to 2-mm layer of low signal intensity that is contiguous with the muscularis. Below the level of the lowermost fibers of the internal sphincter, the anal canal forms the vertical columns of Morgagni, marking the junction between columnar and squamous epithelium (**Fig. 4**).

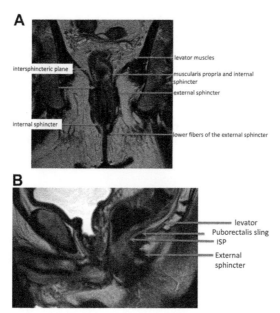

Fig. 3. (*A*) The continuity of the muscularis propria and internal sphincter is well depicted on a coronal MRI. The intersphincteric plane that separates internal sphincter form the somatic muscle "sheet" that is contiguous with the external sphincter. (*B*) Sagittal MRI showing the levator muscles attached at the sacrum the most distal fibers of the levator blend with the upper most fibers of the puborectalis muscle. Fibers of the puborectalis sling in turn blend with the external sphincter.

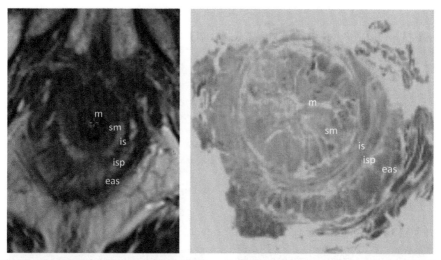

Fig. 4. Anatomy of the anal canal on high resolution MRI with corresponding hematoxylin and eosin histopathology. eas, external anal sphincter; is, internal sphincter; isp, intersphincteric plane; m, mucosa; sm, submucosa

Adjacent Structures

The anatomic hindgut is separated from the anterior visceral compartment by the urogenital septum (a fibromuscular embryonic remnant; **Fig. 5**A). Inferiorly, the horizontal fibers of the transverse perineal muscle separate the anal canal from the urethra in females (**Fig. 5**B) and the crus of the penile bulb in males. More superior, the septum separates the anal canal wall from the apex of prostate and distal vagina in males and females respectively. Laterally, the obturator internus muscles are separated from the lower anal canal by the ischioanal fossa containing fat and the lymphatics and vascular branch supply and drainage to the external sphincter complex.

STAGING

Staging of anal canal cancers follows the American Joint Committee on Cancer/Union Internationale Contre le Cancer system and is determined by size of the primary tumor, presence of local invasion, presence of regional lymphadenopathy, and presence of metastatic disease (**Table 1**).[19] In a study of 19,199 patients with anal carcinoma diagnosed between 1985 and 2000, 25.3% were stage I, 51.8% were stage II, 17.1% were stage III, and 5.7% were stage IV at the time of diagnosis.[20] Staging clearly impacts necessary treatment and prognosis in this tumor type.

IMPACT OF IMAGING ON STAGING OF ANAL CANAL CANCER
Primary Anal Cancer Staging by Imaging

Primary invasive anal cancer is readily depicted on high-resolution MRI as an intermediate signal intensity mass. Most commonly, as with rectal adenocarcinoma, these lesions tend to present as annular or semiannular infiltrating mass lesions and arise within the anal canal (**Fig. 6**A). On occasion, squamous cell carcinoma presents higher and above the anorectal junction, but the TNM classification for squamous cell carcinoma is still used. This separates prognosis according to the maximum length of the tumor. It was originally derived for classification of tumor length by digital rectal examination, but the advent of high-resolution MRI has made it easier to provide objective

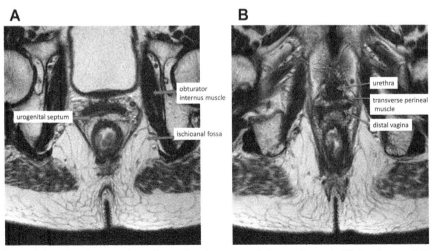

Fig. 5. (A) Embryology and resultant development of the anal canal. (B) Anatomy of the female anal canal.

Table 1
Staging of anal canal cancer

AJCC Stage	Primary Tumor (T) Stage	Lymph Node Status (N)	Distant Metastasis (M)
I	T1	N0	M0
II	T2	N0	M0
	T3	N0	M0
IIIA	T1	N1	M0
	T2	N1	M0
	T3	N1	M0
	T4	N0	M0
IIIB	T4	N1	M0
	Any T	N2	M0
	Any T	N3	M0
IV	Any T	Any N	M1

Primary tumor staging of anal canal cancer: T1: ≤2 cm in greatest dimension, T2: 2 < tumor <5 cm in greatest dimension, T3: >5 cm in greatest dimension, T4: tumor that invades adjacent organs (vagina, urethra, bladder, prostate).

Nodal staging of anal canal cancer: N0: no regional lymph node metastasis, N1: metastasis in perirectal lymph node(s), N2: metastasis in unilateral internal iliac and/or inguinal lymph node(s), N3: metastasis in perirectal and inguinal lymph nodes and/or bilateral internal iliac and/or inguinal lymph nodes.

Distant Metastatic Staging of Anal Canal Cancer: M0: no distant metastasis, M1: distant metastasis.

Abbreviation: AJCC, American Joint Committee on Cancer.

Used with permission of the American Joint Committee on Cancer (AJCC), Chicago, Illinois. The original and primary source for this information is the AJCC Cancer Staging Manual, Seventh Edition (2010) published by Springer Science+Business Media.

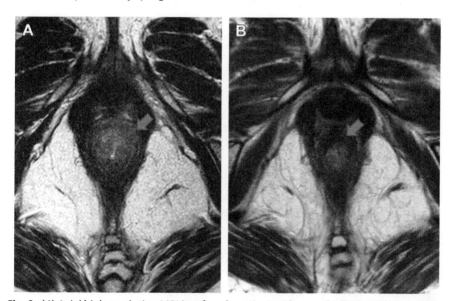

Fig. 6. (*A*) Axial high-resolution MRI in a female patient with a newly diagnosed anal cancer. The primary tumor is seen as a semiannular mass of higher signal intensity (*arrow*) than the anal sphincter and occupies the anterior quadrant. There is extramural spread of 11 mm at the 2 o'clock position which infiltrates inner fibers of left puborectalis and posterior wall of the vagina. (*B*) After chemoradiotherapy, the treated tumor/scar is present in the anterior quadrant (*arrow*). There is no longer any abnormal intermediate signal intensity to indicate residual active tumor and the sphincter anatomic layers, puborectalis and vagina show no evidence of disruption by tumor signal.

measurement. Because chemoradiotherapy is the mainstay of treatment, an accurate anatomic depiction of the radial as well as craniocaudal extent of tumor enables optimal radiotherapy planning and permits a baseline series of imaging for comparison with posttreatment scans to verify response and to monitor the treated tumor and nodal deposits for any suspected recurrence (**Fig. 6**B).

Nodal Spread of Anal Canal Cancer

Nodal spread in anal cancer can be challenging, particularly if perianal inflammation results in reactive lymphadenopathy. Both benign reactive nodes (**Fig. 7**A) and malignant nodes (**Fig. 7**B–D) regress after chemoradiotherapy, and so disappearance of nodes cannot be used as an indicator. Reliance on size criteria is also known to result in overestimation of nodal spread, and the most accurate results are achieved by evaluating the morphologic characteristics that are associated with metastatic infiltration. Nodal infiltration by tumor can result in a breach of the normally smooth lymph node capsule, leading to spiculated irregularity of the node border. Squamous cell infiltration in nodes is often associated with necrosis, which will result in focal high signal intensity within the node giving rise to mixed signal intensity characteristics. Inguinal nodal enlargement is a frequent finding but not always related to malignancy, so targeted ultrasound guided fine needle aspiration of inguinal nodes is a helpful and relatively straightforward means of determining the inguinal nodal status. MRI assessment should include high resolution evaluation of the mesorectal nodes up to the L5/S1 level, the inguinal nodal territory and the external, obturator fossa, internal iliac nodes and common iliac nodes. These are all classified as locoregional lymph nodes but the N stage grouping depends on the sites of nodal spread.

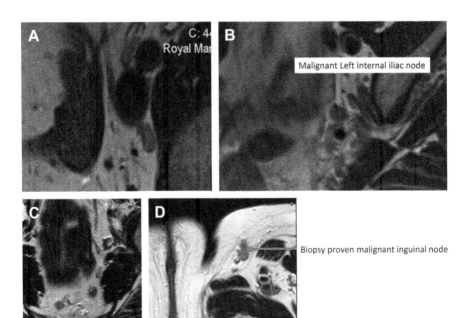

Fig. 7. (A) Benign reactive lymph nodes. (B) Malignant left internal inguinal lymph node (*arrow*). (C) Malignant mesorectal lymph node characterized by nodal capsule irregularity (*arrow*). (D) Biopsy-proven malignant inguinal lymph node.

IMAGING CHARACTERISTICS OF CLINICAL OUTCOMES
Imaging Appearances After Treatment

Traditional imaging has been undertaken at 3 months from the completion of chemoradiotherapy, when treatment related fibrosis established and the low signal intensity of fibrosis can be more readily distinguished from the intermediate signal intensity of residual tumor (**Fig. 8**A). It is now recognized that anal cancers may continue to regress after this initial 3-month assessment, and the majority should have fully regressed by 6 months after completion of treatment. The vast majority of tumors respond fully to treatment and require surveillance only. In a minority of patients,

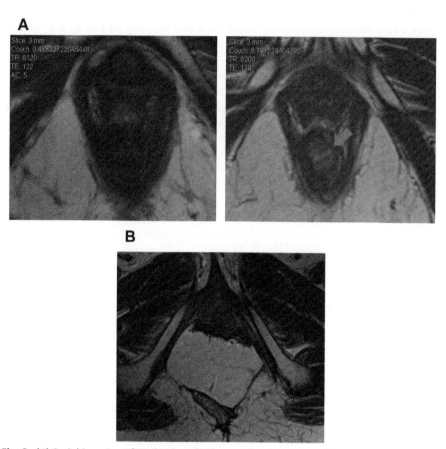

Fig. 8. (A) Serial imaging after chemoradiotherapy for squamous cell carcinoma of the anal canal. The images on the left were undertaken as part of annual follow-up and showed treated tumor as demonstrated by a crescentic low signal scar visible at the level of the puborectalis in the anterior quadrant. At a surveillance scan the following year, the low signal intensity scar was no longer visible; there was instead marked thickening and new intermediate signal along the anterior quadrant of the anal canal. The recurrent tumor was infiltrating the muscularis propria but did not extend into the posterior vaginal wall (arrow). (B) Postoperative appearance of the anal canal after the patient's surgical excision and flap reconstruction. Histology showed an anterior quadrant ulcerated invasive moderately differentiated squamous cell carcinoma that was present at the anorectal junction. The tumor was present in the submucosa and the muscularis propria but did not extend into the levators or the attached vaginal wall.

the tumor fails to regress and in those instances salvage surgery is required to render the patient disease free. The close proximity of neighboring viscera (prostate, urethra, and vagina) means that radical exenterative surgery with or without radical nodal dissection may be necessary.

Imaging Features of the Pelvis During Surveillance

The combination of clinical follow-up assessment, serial imaging, and careful comparison with the initial posttreatment baseline has enabled the earlier diagnosis of recurrence and the consequent radical salvage of pelvic recurrence (see **Fig. 8**). Recurrence within the treated scar can be seen as reemergence of intermediate signal intensity in or around the tumor scar. Emergence of new or progressively enlarging nodes is also readily diagnosed on surveillance MRI and may be treated with radical intent. Imaging is also helpful in the diagnosis of some of treatment related complications, such as fistula formation and insufficiency fracture.

SUMMARY

Anal canal cancer is a tumor type that depends on accurate anatomic staging for optimal treatment planning and cure. In addition to standard diagnostic procedures, including history and physical, laboratory assessment, and endoscopy, modern radiologic imaging techniques are extremely helpful in the assessment of this cancer. The use of multiple robust radiographic modalities has improved staging, response evaluation, and surveillance of this cancer.

REFERENCES

1. Parkin DM. The global health burden of infection-associated cancers in the year 2002. Int J Cancer 2006;118(12):3030–44.
2. Morgan CN, Thompson HR. Surgical anatomy of the anal canal with special reference to the surgical importance of the internal sphincter and conjoint longitudinal muscle. Ann R Coll Surg Engl 1956;19(2):88–114.
3. Kaur H, Choi H, You YN, et al. MR imaging for preoperative evaluation of primary rectal cancer: practical considerations. Radiographics 2012;32(2):389–409.
4. Bamba Y, Itabashi M, Kameoka S. Preoperative evaluation of the depth of anal canal invasion in very low rectal cancer by magnetic resonance imaging and surgical indications for intersphincteric resection. Surg Today 2012;42(4):328–33.
5. Miller EJ, Quan SH, Thaler HT. Treatment of squamous cell carcinoma of the anal canal. Cancer 1991;67(8):2038–41.
6. Leichman LP, Cummings BJ. Anal carcinoma. Curr Probl Cancer 1990;14(3):117–59.
7. Shridhar R, Shibata D, Chan E, et al. Anal cancer: current standards in care and recent changes in practice. CA Cancer J Clin 2015;65(2):139–62.
8. Wells JS, Holstad MM, Thomas T, et al. An integrative review of guidelines for anal cancer screening in HIV-infected persons. AIDS Patient Care STDS 2014;28(7):350–7.
9. Steele SR, Varma MG, Melton GB, et al. Practice parameters for anal squamous neoplasms. Dis Colon Rectum 2012;55(7):735–49.
10. Jacopo M. Endoanal ultrasound for anal cancer staging. Int J colorectal Dis 2011;26(3):385–6.
11. Giovannini M, Bardou VJ, Barclay R, et al. Anal carcinoma: prognostic value of endorectal ultrasound (ERUS). Results of a prospective multicenter study. Endoscopy 2001;33(3):231–6.

12. Otto SD, Lee L, Buhr HJ, et al. Staging anal cancer: prospective comparison of transanal endoscopic ultrasound and magnetic resonance imaging. J Gastrointest Surg 2009;13(7):1292–8.
13. MERCURY Study Group. Extramural depth of tumor invasion at thin-section MR in patients with rectal cancer: results of the MERCURY study. Radiology 2007; 243(1):132–9.
14. Brown G, Richards CJ, Bourne MW, et al. Morphologic predictors of lymph node status in rectal cancer with use of high-spatial-resolution MR imaging with histopathologic comparison. Radiology 2003;227(2):371–7.
15. Trautmann TG, Zuger JH. Positron emission tomography for pretreatment staging and posttreatment evaluation in cancer of the anal canal. Mol Imaging Biol 2005; 7(4):309–13.
16. Cotter SE, Grigsby PW, Siegel BA, et al. FDG-PET/CT in the evaluation of anal carcinoma. Int J Radiat Oncol Biol Phys 2006;65(3):720–5.
17. Deantonio L, Milia ME, Cena T, et al. Anal cancer FDG-PET standard uptake value: correlation with tumor characteristics, treatment response and survival. Radiol Med 2016;121(1):54–9.
18. Caldarella C, Annunziata S, Treglia G, et al. Diagnostic performance of positron emission tomography/computed tomography using fluorine-18 fluorodeoxyglucose in detecting locoregional nodal involvement in patients with anal canal cancer: a systematic review and meta-analysis. ScientificWorldJournal 2014;2014: 196068.
19. Edge SB, Compton CC. AJCC cancer staging manual. New York: Springer; 2010. p. 165–73.
20. Bilimoria KY, Bentrem DJ, Rock CE, et al. Outcomes and prognostic factors for squamous-cell carcinoma of the anal canal: analysis of patients from the National Cancer Data Base. Dis Colon Rectum 2009;52(4):624–31.

Pathology of Anal Cancer

Paulo M. Hoff, MD, PhD[a], Renata Coudry, MD, PhD[b],
Camila Motta Venchiarutti Moniz, MD[a],*

KEYWORDS

- Anal cancer • Anal squamous intraepithelial neoplasia • Squamous cell carcinoma
- Human papilloma virus (HPV) • Molecular

KEY POINTS

- Anal cancer is an uncommon tumor, squamous cell carcinoma (SCC) being the most frequent histology corresponding to 80% of all cases.
- Human papilloma virus (HPV) infection plays a key role in anal cancer development, encoding at least three oncoproteins with stimulatory properties.
- SCC expresses CK5/6, CK 13/19, and p63. P16 is a surrogate marker for the presence of HPV genome in tumor cells.

INTRODUCTION

Anal cancer accounts for approximately 2.4% of gastrointestinal malignancies.[1] Although anal cancer is a rare tumor, its frequency is increasing, especially in high-risk groups.[2] Tumors in this location are generally classified as anal canal or anal margin.

Squamous cell carcinoma (SCC) is the predominant type of tumor and shares many features with cervical cancer. Oncogenic human papilloma virus (HPV) infection plays a major role in both tumors.[3] HIV infection is associated with a higher frequency of HPV-associated premalignant lesions and invasive tumors.[4]

Normal Anatomy of the Anus

The anal canal is the terminal part of the large intestine and is slightly longer in male than in female patients. It measures approximately 4 cm and extends from the rectal ampulla (pelvic floor level) to the anal verge, which is defined as the outer opening of the gastrointestinal tract. The anal verge is at the level of the squamous-mucocutaneous junction with the perianal skin.[5,6]

The authors have nothing to disclose.
[a] Instituto do Câncer do Estado de São Paulo, Faculdade de Medicina da Universidade de São Paulo, São Paulo, São Paulo 01246 000, Brazil; [b] Hospital Sírio Libânes, Rua Dona Adma Jafet, 115 - Bela Vista, São Paulo, São Paulo 01308 050, Brasil
* Corresponding author.
E-mail address: camila_med33@yahoo.com.br

The dentate line (also called pectinate) consists of the anal valves and bases of the anal columns. It represents the anatomic division of the rectum from the anal canal. The dentate line originates from the embryonic union of the ectoderm with the endoderm. The anal canal epithelium can be divided into three zones (**Fig. 1**). The upper part consists of colorectal mucosal type, followed by an anal transition zone (ATZ) that is composed of specialized epithelium that starts at the dentate line and extends from 0.5-1 cm. Finally, the distal anal canal consists of squamous epithelium, which may be partially keratinized.[5,6] The anatomic distribution is clinically significant because it is related to lymphatic drainage and different types of precursor epithelium.

The tumor can be accessed for biopsy using anoscopy, rectoscopy, or direct examination of anal and perineal exophytic lesions.

Histology Classification

Tumors of the anal canal were classified by the World Health Organization (WHO) in three main groups: epithelial, mesenchymal, and secondary tumors. Epithelial tumors were subdivided into malignant and premalignant lesions (**Box 1**).[5]

Human Papilloma Virus Infection

Evidence indicates an association between oncogenic HPV infection with premalignant and malignant lesions of the genital tract, including the anus.[7] The presence of HPV in anal cancer is variable and may be influenced by the methodology used for virus identification and by population characteristics. The HPV infection can be detected in tumor tissue using different techniques, including in situ hybridization (**Fig. 2**) and polymerase chain reaction (PCR).

Currently, 88% of anal SCC tumor samples are usually HPV positive, with different rates according to geographic location.[8] HPV16 infection is the most common, present in 86% of cases. In some cases, coinfection was found with multiple HPV types.[9]

HPV is a nonenveloped virus with double-stranded DNA in circular form, containing a genome of around 8000 base pairs.[7] HPV can remain housed in the nuclei of basal epithelial cells for decades after initial infection of the mucosa, which usually occurs through sexual contact.[10] There are more than 240 types described and the alpha human papillomavirus is usually related to mucosal infection.[11] The high-risk HPV genotypes (16 and 18) encode at least 3 oncoproteins with stimulatory properties: E5, E6,

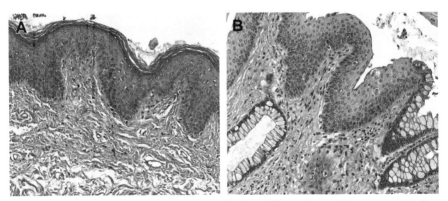

Fig. 1. Normal epithelium. (*A*) Squamous epithelium. (*B*) Anal transition zone epithelium showing in the left cuboidal or polygonal surface cells. In the right can be viewed colonic mucosa with an underlying crypt.

Box 1
World Health Organization histologic classification of tumors of the anal canal

- Epithelial tumors
  - Premalignant lesions
    - Anal intraepithelial neoplasia (dysplasia), low-grade
    - Anal intraepithelial neoplasia (dysplasia), high-grade
    - Bowen disease
    - Perianal squamous intraepithelial neoplasia
    - Paget disease
  - Carcinoma
    - SCC
    - Verrucous carcinoma
    - Undifferentiated carcinoma
    - Adenocarcinoma
    - Mucinous adenocarcinoma
  - Neuroendocrine neoplasms
    - Neuroendocrine tumor (NET)
      - NET G1 (carcinoid)
      - NET G2
    - Neuroendocrine carcinoma (NEC)
      - Small cell NEC
      - Large cell NEC
    - Mixed adenoneuroendocrine carcinoma

- Mesenchymal tumors

- Secondary tumors

From Bosman FT, Carneiro F, Hruban RH, et al. WHO Classification of Tumours of the Digestive System, Fourth Edition. Lyon: IARC Press, 2010. p. 184; with permission.

---

and E7. Integration of the viral DNA in the genome of the host cell is important for the progression of preneoplastic lesions to invasive carcinoma. During HPV integration, breakage of the E2 region of the viral genome occurs in the DNA of the infected cells, which causes the loss of suppressor function of the E2 protein. This results in an increased expression of the E6 and E7 proteins and their stimulation promotes invasiveness and keratinocyte immortalization.[10] E6 and E7 expression is required for the induction and maintenance of the transformed state of HPV-related neoplasm. The protein E7 interacts with Rb protein (pRb) and E6 is able to bind and inactivate P53.[12]

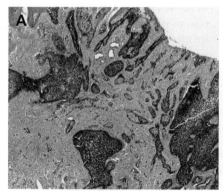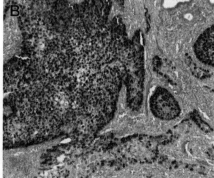

Fig. 2. In situ hybridization. (*A*) Note the positivity for high-risk HPV probe. (*B*) Diffuse staining with condensed and uniform signs in the nuclei of the cancer cells.

PREINVASIVE LESIONS

There are different terminologies used to describe premalignant lesions of the anal region. Squamous lesions were first described in the anal margin 50 years ago and they were initially classified as cutaneous lesions, such as Bowen disease and carcinoma in situ. Over time, a causal relationship was established between anal dysplasia and HPV perianal infection. However, terminologies of squamous precancerous lesions of anal canal continued to be diverse. The WHO classification (**Box 1**), for instance, has four items related to premalignant squamous lesions. There are two items grading intraepithelial neoplasia/dysplasia in low and high grade. In addition, two other categories, Bowen disease, and perianal squamous intraepithelial neoplasia. These last two probably designating the same lesion. To make things even more complicated, the American Joint Committee on Cancer (AJCC) definition for primary tumors classifies noninvasive squamous lesions as carcinoma in situ, Bowen disease, high-grade squamous intraepithelial lesion (HSIL), and anal intraepithelial neoplasias (AIN) 2-3. This shows the need to propose a clearer classification so that the work of clinicians and pathologists is more uniform.

Squamous Intraepithelial Lesions

Because HPV plays a causal role in perianal and anal neoplasia, anal squamous precancerous lesions should now be classified according to the same criteria and terminology as their cervical counterparts using the Lower Anogenital Squamous Terminology (LAST) system.[3]

A consensus process was organized by the College of American Pathologists and the American Society for Colposcopy and Cervical Pathology to recommend terminology unified across lower anogenital sites. The aim of this system of standardization was to create uniformity in histologic nomenclature for HPV-associated tumors that occurred in the anogenital tract. This permits a better use of current biomarkers and enables an efficient communication between specialties that establish the diagnosis and treatment of these lesions. The recommendation for classifying preinvasive lesions in the anal canal was similar to the cervical site. Hence, the same two-tiered nomenclature of intraepithelial lesion could be applied: low-grade squamous intraepithelial lesion (LSIL) and HSIL. The lesions are located above the basement membrane and may originate from the transitional or squamous epithelium of the anal canal. In the LAST system, condyloma is located with LSIL in the same category and Bowenoid papulosis is considered a special form of HSIL. Besides this, it does not discriminate cytologic from tissue specimens. Therefore, the terms LSIL and HSIL can be used in both materials. However, for histopathological diagnosis, the suffix AIN can be used; therefore, the lesion in the anal canal can be subcategorized as: LSIL-AIN 1 and HSIL-AIN 2-3.

LSIL-AIN 1 can be defined as a proliferation of metaplastic squamous cells with nuclear atypia in the lower third of the epithelium or demonstrating koilocytotic changes in a papillary lesion (**Fig. 3**). The histologic findings of HSIL-AIN 2-3 consist of a thickened proliferating epithelium containing atypical cells showing abnormal nuclear polarity, nuclear pleomorphism, and high nuclear hyperchromatism: cytoplasmic ratio and increased mitotic activity (**Fig. 4**).[5]

To date, knowledge of the long-term natural history of anal squamous intraepithelial lesion is still not well established. It is postulated that anal LSIL, corresponding to AIN 1, spontaneously regresses but may also progress to HSIL.[13] The overall progression rate of HSIL, corresponding to HSIL-AIN grade 2 or 3 invasive carcinoma, is 2% to 9% but can reach 50% in immunocompromised individuals (**Fig. 5**).[14]

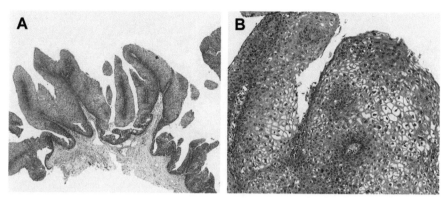

Fig. 3. Condyloma. (*A*) Note the exophytic polypoid feature with minimal stromal proliferation. Condyloma is equivalent to LSIL and AIN 1. (*B*) Enlarged nuclei and koilocytotic atypia.

Paget Disease

Primary anal Paget disease has a cutaneous origin and affects areas densely populated by apocrine glands arising from adnexal stem cells. Malignant cells produce mucus and infiltrate all layers of the epidermis. Histology reveals large cells with plentiful pale cytoplasm and large nuclei, and sometimes the tumor cells acquire a signet ring appearance.[5,15]

MALIGNANT NEOPLASMS

Even though cancer of the anal canal is rare, a variety of malignant neoplasms involve tumors in this location. Almost all of these are SCC. Other rare anal canal neoplasms include adenocarcinoma, neuroendocrine tumors, malignant melanoma, lymphomas, and various mesenchymal tumors.

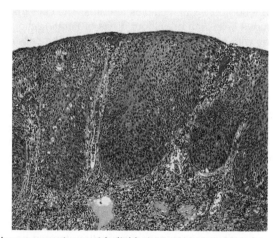

Fig. 4. High-grade squamous intraepithelial lesion–AIN 3. Note the abnormal basaloid cells having an increased nuclear cytoplasmic ratio extending to the entire thickness of the epithelium but restricted to the basement membrane.

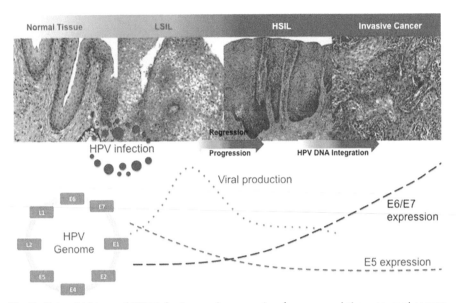

Fig. 5. Natural history of HPV infection and progression from normal tissue to anal cancer. Progressive changes in squamous epithelium through loss of normal apoptotic cell mechanism due to the presence of E6 and E7 oncoproteins. In SCC, virus genome integration occurs with loss of E2 regulatory region, resulting in uncontrolled E6/E7, p53, and pRb production.

Squamous Cell Carcinoma

This is the most common histology of anal cancer, corresponding to 80%.[16] The histologic classification of anal SCC was previously considered a complex issue, with several subtypes using a variable terminology. The current WHO classification recommends that the generic term SCC should be used for all squamous malignancies of the anal canal.[5] Tumors located in the anal canal predominantly develop at the transformation zone between the squamous and columnar epithelium of the anal canal[14]; and most tumors are composed of multiples features. The cells may have large pale eosinophilic squamous cells with or without areas of keratinization. Another pattern is tumor-cell islands with prominent palisading of nuclei. The cells can constitute tumor nests and differentiated tumors may present peripheral palisading or central keratinization.[5,15]

In the past, the basaloid subtype, also called cloacogenic carcinoma, was included in the WHO classification. It was withdrawn because either it was difficult to reproduce this diagnosis and prognosis, or the SCC treatment lacked correlation. Currently, the use of SCC is recommended to describe the main diagnosis, with a comment detailing particularities of each sample as a degree of differentiation, such as presence of mucinous, basaloid features and degree of keratinization (**Fig. 6**).[5]

STAGING

Two distinct categories of tumors arise in the anal canal region. Those that develop from the mucosa, called the anal canal tumors, and tumors that arise within the skin at or distal to the squamous mucocutaneous junction, termed as perianal cancers. This last type of tumor is staged and treated as skin cancer and not like anal canal cancer.[17] Staging of anal carcinomas should be determined in agreement with the criteria

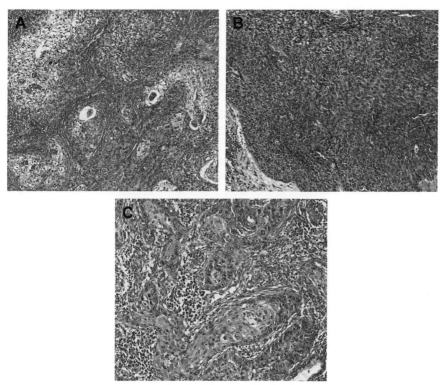

Fig. 6. SCC. (*A*) Note the clear cell features and abnormal keratinization. (*B*) The tumor shows basaloid features. (C) Nests infiltrated by keratinization.

of the AJCC (**Tables 1** and **2**).[17] Because most cases of anal cancer are treated using nonsurgical procedures, the role of staging based on the histopathological evaluation is limited to cases of resection in an early stage, salvage surgical treatment or sentinel lymph node procedure.[18]

Verrucous Carcinoma

The Buschke-Löwenstein tumor, or giant malignant condyloma, is an intermediate variant between condyloma and SCC. This tumor often presents as a large mass with cauliflower appearance and has an endophytic and exophytic growth. The lesion size can range from 1 to 30 cm and can initiate in the perianal skin, anal canal, or distal rectum.[19] Despite a benign histologic appearance with acanthosis and papillomatosis in regular arrangement of the epithelial layers, this tumor may present a locally destructive behavior by direct deeper invasion.[5]

Adenocarcinoma

This tumor can originate in the mucosa, anal glands, or anal canal fistulae, and may appear near the anal duct as a small pedunculated or ulcerated lesion,[15] or produce a submucosal mass. An association with Paget and Crohn disease is described. Generally, adenocarcinomas associated with congenital or acquired fistulae are mucin productive.

Table 1
Tumor-nodes-metastasis staging anal cancer

Primary tumor (T)

TX	Primary tumor cannot be assessed
T0	No evidence of primary tumor
Tis	Carcinoma in situ Bowen disease, high-grade squamous intraepithelial lesion (HSIL), anal intraepithelial neoplasia 2–3 (AIN 2–3)
T1	Tumor 2 cm or less in greatest dimension
T2	Tumor more than 2 cm but not more than 5 cm in greatest dimension
T3	Tumor more than 5 cm in greatest dimension
T4	Tumor of any size invades adjacent organs; for example, vagina, urethra, bladder[a]

Regional lymph nodes (N)

NX	Regional lymph nodes cannot be assessed
N0	No regional lymph node metastasis
N1	Metastasis in perirectal lymph nodes
N2	Metastasis in unilateral internal iliac and/or inguinal lymph nodes
N3	Metastasis in perirectal and inguinal lymph nodes and/or bilateral internal iliac and/or inguinal lymph nodes

Distant metastasis (M)

M0	No distant metastasis
M1	Distant metastasis

[a] Direct invasion of the rectal wall, perirectal skin, subcutaneous tissue, or the sphincter muscles is not classified as T4.

From Edge SB, Compton CC, Fritz AG, et al. Cancer Staging Manual. 7th edition. New York, Dordrecht, Heidelberg, London: Springer; 2010. p. 167; with permission.

Table 2
Anatomic stage: prognostic groups

	Tumor (T)	Node (N)	Metastasis (M)
0	Tis	N0	M0
I	T1	N0	M0
II	T2	N0	M0
	T3	N0	M0
IIIA	T1	N1	M0
	T2	N1	M0
	T3	N1	M0
	T4	N0	M0
IIIB	T4	N1	M0
	Any T	N2	M0
	Any T	N3	M0
IV	Any T	Any N	M1

From Edge SB, Compton CC, Fritz AG, et al. Cancer Staging Manual. 7th Edition. New York, Dordrecht, Heidelberg, London: Springer; 2010. p. 165; with permission.

OTHER TUMOR TYPES

A variety of other tumor types may arise less frequently in the anal canal and make recognition more difficult.

Melanoma

Anal melanomas are a rare disease and account for 1% of anal and perianal lesions.[15] Two-thirds are found as pigmented lesions, usually ulcerated and bleeding. Similar to melanomas that arise in other mucous membranes, they are generally of the acrolentiginous type. Retrospective studies have reported poor prognosis, especially in patients with lymph node involvement or metastasis at diagnosis. Anal melanoma presents the same histologic appearance as that of cutaneous melanoma with S-100 expression. Positive c-kit was reported in 45%.[15,20] Differential diagnosis of Paget anal melanoma can be difficult if based solely on histologic features; therefore, association with immunohistochemical evaluation is useful.

Mesenchymal Tumors

Uncommonly lipomas, hemangiomas, leiomyomas and leiomyosarcomas, rhabdomyosarcomas, granular cell tumors, and Kaposi sarcoma may be located in the anal and perianal region.[5,15]

Basal Cell Carcinoma of the Anus

Basal cell carcinoma comprises 0.2% of anorectal neoplasms[21] and affects the skin of the anal region. There is no evidence of the carcinogenic role of HPV in this tumor but SCC with basaloid features may show overlapping of histologic findings with basal cell carcinoma.[5,21] Both tumors may have nests of oval cells with moderate quantity of eosinophilic to basophilic cytoplasm, peripheral nuclear palisading, and assorted mitotic activity. In a retrospective study of basal cell carcinoma, the nodular subtype of basal cell carcinoma was the most frequent and this tumor presented more retraction artifact and no atypical mitotic figures.[21]

Neuroendocrine Tumors

Anal neuroendocrine tumors are unusual and account for 1% of all anal cancers.[22] Anal small cell carcinoma has poor prognosis and generally begins in the upper part of the anal canal, grows fast, and promotes metastasis. Histologically, it may be confused with SCC due to basaloid features but immunohistochemistry is an important tool for differential diagnosis. Small cell carcinoma usually demonstrates positive chromogranin, leu7, neuron-specific enolase, synaptophysin, and neurofilament protein.[15]

Undifferentiated Tumors

These tumors do not have the characteristics that allow them to be classified as squamous or glandular. They usually have a high mitotic index and aggressive behavior.[15]

Secondary Tumors

Metastasis in the anal canal is extremely rare. Rectal and retrorectal cancer (chordomas, chondrosarcomas, and neurogenic tumors) can extend and invade the anus.[5,15]

IMMUNOHISTOCHEMISTRY OF ANAL CANAL CANCER

SCC expresses CK5/6, CK 13/19, and p63. CK7 is positive in adenocarcinoma and generally absent in SCC but tumors with adenoid cystic pattern can be CK7+. Classic

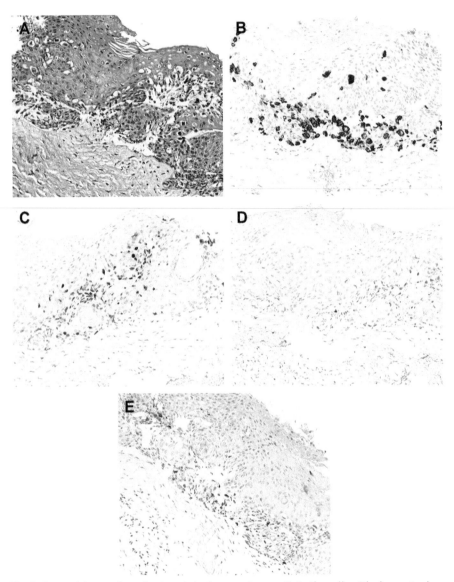

Fig. 7. Pagetoid extension of colorectal adenocarcinoma. Note the cells with clear cytoplasm within the squamous epithelium (*A*). These cells are positive for CK20 (*B*), Positive for CDX-2 (*C*), negative for GCDFP-15 (*D*), and negative for HMB45 immunostaining (*E*).

neuroendocrine markers are positive for neuroendocrine tumors, melanocytic markers for melanomas, and a panel of lymphoid markers for lymphomas. Primary perianal Paget disease is positive for CK and gross cystic disease fluid protein 15 (GCDFP15). However, when associated with a pagetoid extension of colorectal or urothelial adenocarcinoma, the pagetoid cells tend to coexpress CK20 and lack GCDFP-15 (**Fig. 7**).[23] The main differential diagnoses of anal canal tumors are summarized in **Box 1**.[5,15]

p16

In quiescent cells, pRb is active in the hypophosphorylated form. In its active form, it is able to bind and sequester E2F family transcription factors. The free form of E2F can stimulate activity of gene promoters that coordinate cell cycle transition from GAP (G)-1 to synthesis (S). In this way, active pRb is able to block cell cycle progression.[24,25]

The phosphorylation of pRb by cyclin dependent kinase (CDK) reduces its affinity for E2F factors and leads to cell cycle progression.[24,25] The CDKN2 is a tumor suppressor gene and encodes p16 protein (also called CDKN2A) that actively participates in the cell cycle, blocking activity of CDK involved in pRb phosphorylation. p16 expression is normally repressed by pRb-E2F complex but this process is inhibited by the presence of viral HPV E7 protein. Presence of p16 evaluated by immunohistochemistry is a surrogate marker for the presence of HPV genome in tumor cells in cervical and head and neck cancer.[26]

In SCC, p16 immunohistochemistry expression has shown better prognosis in retrospective series; however, these data need to be further investigated in larger prospective studies.[9,27] Besides this, p16 protein is a useful marker to confirm a diagnosis of HPV-related anal HSIL (**Fig. 8, Table 3**).[16]

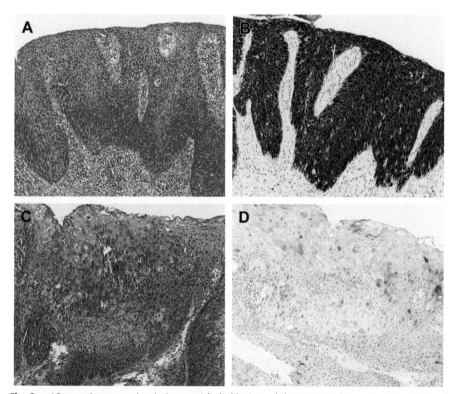

Fig. 8. p16 protein expression in intraepithelial lesions. (*A*) Hematoxylin-eosin stain (H&E) of HSIL-AIN3. Note the p16 immunostaining extending to the entire epithelial thickness (*B*). LSIL-AIN1 (*C*), note a mottled focal p16 expression (*D*), considering this case as a negative staining. This result argues against the diagnosis of HSIL (AIN 2-3).

Table 3
Immunohistochemistry of anal canal tumors

	SCC	Anal Gland Adenocarcinoma	Paget (Primary)	Paget (Secondary)	Melanoma	Neuroendocrine	Basal Cell Carcinoma
CK5/6	+	−	−	−	−	−	+
CK7/20	−/−	+/usually−	+/−	usually−/+	−	−/−	−/−
AE1/AE2	+	+	+	+	−	+	+
CAM5.2	+	+	+	+	−	+	…
GCDFP-15	−	−	+	−	−	−	−
CDX-2	−	usually−	−	+	−	−	−
CEA	−	−	+	+	−	−	−
Mucin	−	+	+	+	−	−	−
HMB45	−	−	−	−	+	−	−
MELAN-A	−	−	−	−	+	−	−
Vimentin	−	−	−	−	+	−	−
S100	−	−	−	−	+	−	−
Ber-EP4	−	+	+	+	−	−	+
p63	+	−	−	−	−	−	+
Chromogranin	−	−	−	−	−	+	−
Synaptophysin	−	−	−	−	−	+	−

Abbreviations: AE1/AE3, anti-pan cytokeratin [AE1/AE3]; Ber-EP4, anti-epithelial cell adhesion antibody [Ber-EP4]; CAM5.2, anticytokeratin [CAM5.2]; CDX2, caudal type homeobox 2; CEA, carcinoembryonic antigen; CK, cytokeratin; GCDFP-15, gross cystic disease fluid protein-15; HMB45, antimelanoma antibody (clone HMB45); MELAN-A, product of the MART-1 gene (recognized by antibody 103); p63, 63 protein; S-100, S-100 protein.

MOLECULAR FEATURES OF ANAL CANAL CANCER

There is paucity of data regarding the molecular profile of anal canal cancer due to the rarity of this disease. Genomic instability is important in cell transformation process and recognized as a risk factor for cancer development. Genetic aberrations in key genes can help tumor cells to obtain selective advantages and have demonstrated that HPV infection might increase DNA damage, endogenous mutations, and chromosome gain.

Recent studies have detected gain in chromosome 3q. In a study on 52 subjects with SCC or anal dysplasia, the gain in chromosome 3q in *PIK3CA* loci was frequent in high-grade dysplasia (53%) and cancer samples (78%) but was not seen in low-grade dysplasia or normal tissue, suggesting a possible involvement of this gene in the pathogenesis and progression of SCC.[28,29] Mutations in the *PIK3CA* gene in tumor samples are also described in retrospectives studies with variable frequency varying from 4% to 32%.[30–33] Discovered in the 1980s, the dimeric enzyme kinase lipid family, called phosphoinositide 3-kinases (PI3Ks), participates in regulating cellular functions such as survival, proliferation and differentiation.[34] Other studies reported chromosomal loses in 11q, 3p, 4p, 13q, 17p, 5p, and 18q.[35]

Mutations in the *EGFR*, *KRAS*, and *BRAF* genes are rare in SCC. Presence of *KRAS* mutations was described in 0% to 4%,[30,32,36–38] *BRAF* in 0% to 4.7%,[30,32,38] and *EGFR* in 0% to 3%.[36,37]

The prognostic role and impact of these mutations on the clinical outcome of SCC patients undergoing curative treatment are still controversial and require further investigation in prospective studies.

REFERENCES

1. Siegel RL, Miller KD, Jemal A. Cancer statistics 2016. CA Cancer J Clin 2016;66: 7–30.
2. Nelson RA, Levine AM, Bernstein L, et al. Changing patterns of anal canal carcinoma in the United States. J Clin Oncol 2013;31(12):1569–75.
3. Darragh TM, Colgan TJ, Cox JT, et al. The Lower Anogenital Squamous Terminology Standardization Project for HPV-Associated lesions: background and consensus recommendations from the College of American Pathologists and the American Society for Colposcopy and Cervical Pathology. Arch Pathol Lab Med 2012;136(10):1266–97.
4. Machalek DA, Poynten M, Jin F, et al. Anal human papillomavirus infection and associated neoplastic lesions in men who have sex with men: a systematic review and meta-analysis. Lancet Oncol 2012;13(5):487–500.
5. Bosman FT, Carneiro F, Hruban RH, et al. WHO classification of tumours of the digestive system. 4th edition. vol. 3. Lyon: International Agency for Research on Cancer; 2010. p. 184–93.
6. Gami B, Kubba F, Ziprin P. Human papilloma virus and squamous cell carcinoma of the anus. Clin Med Insights Oncol 2014;8:113–9.
7. Ostrbenk A, Kocjan BJ, Hosnjak L, et al. Identification of a novel human papillomavirus, type HPV199, isolated from a nasopharynx and anal canal, and complete genomic characterization of papillomavirus species gamma-12. PLoS One 2015;10(9):e0138628.
8. Alemany L, Saunier M, Alvarado-Cabrero I, et al. Human papillomavirus DNA prevalence and type distribution in anal carcinomas worldwide. Int J Cancer 2015;136(1):98–107.

9. Mai S, Welzel G, Ottstadt M, et al. Prognostic relevance of HPV infection and p16 overexpression in squamous cell anal cancer. Int J Radiat Oncol Biol Phys 2015; 93(4):819–27.

10. Hellner K, Munger K. Human papillomaviruses as therapeutic targets in human cancer. J Clin Oncol 2011;29(13):1785–94.

11. Egawa N, Egawa K, Griffin H, et al. Human papillomaviruses; epithelial tropisms, and the development of neoplasia. Viruses 2015;7(7):3863–90.

12. Klingelhutz AJ, Roman A. Cellular transformation by human papillomaviruses: lessons learned by comparing high- and low-risk viruses. Virology 2012;424(2): 77–98.

13. Berry JM, Jay N, Cranston RD, et al. Progression of anal high-grade squamous intraepithelial lesions to invasive anal cancer among HIV-infected men who have sex with men. Int J Cancer 2014;134(5):1147–55.

14. Leeds IL, Fang SH. Anal cancer and intraepithelial neoplasia screening: a review. World J Gastrointest Surg 2016;8(1):41–51.

15. Fenoglio-Preiser CM, Stemmermann GN, Lantz PE, et al. Gastrointestinal pathology: an atlas and text. 3th edition. Philadelphia: Wolters Kluwer/Lippincott Williams & Wilkins; 2008. p. 1067–97.

16. Flejou JF. An update on anal neoplasia. Histopathology 2015;66(1):147–60.

17. Edge SB, Compton CC, Fritz AG, et al. Cancer staging manual. 7th Edition. New York, Dordrecht, Heidelberg, London: Springer; 2010. p. 165–71.

18. Glynne-Jones R, Nilsson PJ, Aschele C, et al. Anal cancer: ESMO-ESSO-ESTRO clinical practice guidelines for diagnosis, treatment and follow-up. Eur J Surg Oncol 2014;40(10):1165–76.

19. Garrett K, Kalady MF. Anal neoplasms. Surg Clin North Am 2010;90(1):147–61 [Table of Contents].

20. Torres-Cabala CA, Wang WL, Trent J, et al. Correlation between KIT expression and KIT mutation in melanoma: a study of 173 cases with emphasis on the acral-lentiginous/mucosal type. Mod Pathol 2009;22(11):1446–56.

21. Patil DT, Goldblum JR, Billings SD. Clinicopathological analysis of basal cell carcinoma of the anal region and its distinction from basaloid squamous cell carcinoma. Mod Pathol 2013;26(10):1382–9.

22. Lee RT, Ferreira J, Friedman K, et al. A rare cause of constipation: obstructing small cell neuroendocrine carcinoma of the anal canal. Int J Colorectal Dis 2015;30(9):1291–2.

23. Dabbs DJ. Diagnostic immunohistochemistry. 3th edition. Philadelphia: Saunders Elsevier; 2010. p. 500–40.

24. Hsieh R, Firmiano A, Sotto MN. Expression of p16 protein in acral lentiginous melanoma. Int J Dermatol 2009;48(12):1303–7.

25. Sherr CJ, Roberts JM. CDK inhibitors: positive and negative regulators of G1-phase progression. Genes Dev 1999;13(12):1501–12.

26. Gilbert DC, Williams A, Allan K, et al. p16INK4A, p53, EGFR expression and KRAS mutation status in squamous cell cancers of the anus: correlation with outcomes following chemo-radiotherapy. Radiother Oncol 2013;109(1):146–51.

27. Yhim HY, Lee NR, Song EK, et al. The prognostic significance of tumor human papillomavirus status for patients with anal squamous cell carcinoma treated with combined chemoradiotherapy. Int J Cancer 2011;129(7):1752–60.

28. Ricciardi R, Burks E, Schoetz DJ, et al. Is there a gain in chromosome 3q in the pathway to anal cancer? Dis Colon Rectum 2014;57(10):1183–7.

29. Liu SV, Lenkiewicz E, Evers L, et al. Genomic analysis and selected molecular pathways in rare cancers. Phys Biol 2012;9(6):065004.

30. Smaglo BG, Tesfaye A, Halfdanarson TR, et al. Comprehensive multiplatform biomarker analysis of 199 anal squamous cell carcinomas. Oncotarget 2015; 6(41):43594–604.
31. Casadei Gardini A, Capelli L, Ulivi P, et al. KRAS, BRAF and PIK3CA status in squamous cell anal carcinoma (SCAC). PLoS One 2014;9(3):e92071.
32. Martin V, Zanellato E, Franzetti-Pellanda A, et al. EGFR, KRAS, BRAF, and PIK3CA characterization in squamous cell anal cancer. Histol Histopathol 2014; 29(4):513–21.
33. Patel H, Polanco-Echeverry G, Segditsas S, et al. Activation of AKT and nuclear accumulation of wild type TP53 and MDM2 in anal squamous cell carcinoma. Int J Cancer 2007;121(12):2668–73.
34. Liu P, Cheng H, Roberts TM, et al. Targeting the phosphoinositide 3-kinase pathway in cancer. Nat Rev Drug Discov 2009;8(8):627–44.
35. Gervaz P, Hirschel B, Morel P. Molecular biology of squamous cell carcinoma of the anus. Br J Surg 2006;93(5):531–8.
36. Van Damme N, Deron P, Van Roy N, et al. Epidermal growth factor receptor and K-RAS status in two cohorts of squamous cell carcinomas. BMC Cancer 2010; 10:189.
37. Paliga A, Onerheim R, Gologan A, et al. EGFR and K-ras gene mutation status in squamous cell anal carcinoma: a role for concurrent radiation and EGFR inhibitors? Br J Cancer 2012;107(11):1864–8.
38. Prigge ES, Urban K, Stiegler S, et al. No evidence of oncogenic KRAS mutations in squamous cell carcinomas of the anogenital tract and head and neck region independent of human papillomavirus and p16(INK4a) status. Hum Pathol 2014;45(11):2347–54.

Treatment of the Primary Tumor in Anal Canal Cancers

Rob Glynne-Jones, FRCR, FRCP[a],*, Sheela Rao, MD, FRCP[b,c]

KEYWORDS

- Squamous cell carcinoma of the anus • Anal carcinoma • Chemotherapy
- Radiotherapy • Chemoradiation • Combined modality • Immunotherapy
- Local recurrence

KEY POINTS

- Squamous cell carcinoma of the anus is generally a localized disease with a relatively low risk of metastatic disease at presentation; thus, local control is the overriding aim of treatment.
- Randomized phase III trials have established the combination of 5-fluorouracil–based chemoradiation concurrent with mitomycin C as the standard of care rather than primary surgery.
- The TNM clinical staging system is based on accurate assessment of size (T stage), regional lymph node involvement, and metastatic spread.
- Assessment and management of anal cancer are best determined by specialist multidisciplinary teams, and treatment should be carried out in specialized centers.
- Future research should attempt to integrate novel biomarker-driven targets, such as anti-CTLA4, anti–programmed cell death, and programmed cell death-ligand 1, into chemoradiation schedules.

INTRODUCTION

Squamous cell carcinoma of the anus (SCCA) is an uncommon malignancy representing approximately 2% of all gastrointestinal malignancies. The incidence has been increasing over the past decade, probably reflecting more widespread infection with the main causal factor human papillomavirus (HPV).

Conflict of Interest Statements: R. Glynne-Jones has received honoraria for lectures and advisory boards and has been supported in attending international meetings by Merck, Pfizer, Sanofi-Aventis, Eli-Lilley, and Roche. He has also received unrestricted grants for research from Merck Serono, Sanofi-Aventis, and Roche. S. Rao has received honoraria for lectures and advisory boards and has been supported in attending international meetings by Merck Serono, Roche, Sanofi-Aventis, Eli Lilly, Servier, Amgen, and Celgene.
[a] Mount Vernon Centre for Cancer Treatment, Rickmansworth Road, Northwood, Middlesex HA6 2RN, UK; [b] Royal Marsden Hospital, London, UK; [c] Royal Marsden Hospital, Downs Road, Sutton, Surrey SM2 5PT, UK
* Corresponding author.
E-mail address: Rob.glynnejones@nhs.net

SCCA is generally a localized disease with a low risk of metastatic disease at presentation. Retrospective studies and randomized trials suggest that locoregional failure is the predominant pattern of relapse,[1–4] usually in the radiotherapy high-dose volume, and often within the first 2 years following completion of chemoradiation (CRT) treatment. Uncontrolled local recurrence is ultimately responsible for most cancer-related deaths, making local control the primary aim of treatment.

Surgical resection was the standard treatment in the 1970s, which involved removal of the anal canal and a permanent stoma. In the past, radiation alone was also often used to treat SCCA using high doses with split-course schedules and interstitial brachytherapy. The pioneering work of Nigro and colleagues[5,6] and subsequent confirmatory studies in the United States highlighted the efficacy of CRT using relatively low doses of fractionated radiotherapy (30–45 Gy) combined with 5-fluorouracil (5-FU) and mitomycin C (MMC). Subsequently, 2 randomized trials[7,8] compared a radiotherapy schedule of 45 Gy boosted with a further 15 to 25 Gy after a gap of 6 weeks against an identical regimen with concurrent 5-FU/MMC. These trials showed radiation alone could result in local control in approximately 45% to 55% of patients. However, both trials confirmed chemoradiotherapy significantly improved outcomes over radiation alone.

Significant toxicity was reported for MMC. So concurrent 5-FU and MMC or 5-FU alone were randomly compared in the CRT component in the RTOG 8704 trial.[9] The addition of MMC significantly improved both disease-free survival (DFS) and colostomy-free survival (CFS).[9] Thus, a series of randomized trials[7–11] all confirmed the efficacy of concurrent CRT with 5-FU/MMC and relegated the role of surgery to salvage of CRT failures. The small Action Clinique Coordonees en Cancerologie Digestive (ACCORD-03) trial, in contrast, used concurrent 5-FU/cisplatin.[12]

The standard of care both in Europe and North America is 5-FU/MMC CRT and is recommended in guidelines.[13,14] This schedule results in complete tumor regression in 80% to 90%, with a high level of permanent disease control particularly for cT1/T2 tumors. The 5-year overall survival (OS) reached 78% in the MMC arm of the RTOG 9811 trial,[15] 71% in the CRT-alone arms without neoadjuvant chemotherapy (NACT) in ACCORD-03,[12] and 79% in the MMC arm of Anal Cancer Trial II (ACT II).[11]

Preservation of sphincter function is usually achieved; but with doses of 50 to 60 Gy, there is a risk of fecal incontinence.[16] In more advanced T3/T4 cancers with nodal metastases, it is more difficult to achieve local control[17]; a substantial proportion of such patients will fail within 2 years. In the ACT II, patients with cT3/T4 cancers and nodal metastases had a 3-year progression-free survival (PFS) of 63%.[11]

Randomized phase III trials by RTOG 9811,[10] the ACCORD-03 phase III trial,[12] and the ACT II trial[11] failed to show any additional benefit in terms of PFS/DFS by increasing the radiotherapy boost dose or replacing MMC with cisplatin during CRT. Additional cisplatin-based chemotherapy given as induction before CRT[10,12] or as maintenance or consolidation after CRT[11] has not improved outcomes (**Table 1**).

SCCA regresses slowly following radiation or CRT. In early trials a 6 to 8 week planned gap between the completion of CRT and a radiotherapy boost allowed the acute toxicity of skin and mucosal surfaces to resolve.[7,8] During this interval the tumor would shrink, and permit an interstitial implant to the smallest possible volume - minimizing the risk of radiation induced necrosis. This strategy also allowed selection of nonresponders for salvage either by dose-escalation of the radiotherapy boost or by surgical resection. Later trials continued this approach although shortened the interval.[10,12] However this practice defied radiobiological principles, because the gap

Table 1
The more recent phase III randomized trials (1998–2008) in squamous cell carcinoma of the anus and their characteristics of the randomized trials comparing different chemoradiation regimens

Trial Name (Years)	Number of Patients	Design	RT Dose	Comparison 1	Comparison 2	Primary End Point
RTOG 9811 (1998–2005) (Ajani et al,[10] 2008)	644	NACT cisplatin/5-FU Then 5-FU/cisplatin/RT (ie, 4 courses) vs 5-FU/MMC/RT	Phase I 45 Gy/25# in 5.0–6.5 wk T3/T4, N+, or residual T2 boost to 54–59 Gy	NACT with 5-FU 1000 mg/m² days 1–4, 29–32, and cisplatin 75 mg/m² then CRT 5-FU/cisplatin vs MMC 10 mg/m² days 1 and 29 and 5-FU 1000 mg/m² days 1–4, 29–32 CRT		DFS
ACCORD-03 (1999–2005) (Peiffert et al,[12] 2012)	307	2 × 2 factorial NACT (5-FU/cisplatin, 2 cycles) vs no NACT Standard vs high-dose boost for responders	Phase I 45 Gy/25#/33 d 3-wk gap then 15-Gy boost standard arms; 20 Gy–25 Gy boost (high-dose arms) for responders; 40% received brachytherapy boost	NACT with 5-FU 800 mg/m² days 1–4, 29–32 and cisplatin 80 g/m² on days 1 and 29; then CRT 5-FU/cisplatin on days as mentioned earlier with RT	Dose escalation of RT boost 15-Gy boost standard arms 20-Gy–25-Gy boost (high-dose arms) for responders	CFS Secondary end points: local control, OS, and cancer-specific survival
ACT II (UKCCCR) (2001–2008) (James et al,[11] 2013)	940	2 × 2 factorial 5-FU/ MMC vs 5-FU cisplatin CRT and consolidation 5-FU/ cisplatin vs control	Phase I 30/6 Gy/17# in 3.5 wk then phase II 19.8 Gy/11# conformal Total 50.4 Gy/28#/38 d no gap	Cisplatin 60 mg/m² d 1 and 29 vs 12 mg/m² MMC day 1 with 5-FU 1000 mg/m² days 1–4, 29–32 CRT	Consolidation 2 courses 5-FU 1000 mg/m² and cisplatin 60 mg/m²	Relapse-free survival

Abbreviations: Cisplatin, cisplatinum; HDRT, high-dose radiotherapy; NS, not significant; OTT, overall treatment time; RT, radiotherapy.

allows the cancer cells to repopulate toward the end of radiotherapy, which in theory partly accounts for treatment failure.[18,19] The only trial that obeyed these constraints and mandated a continuous schedule and prohibited a planned interval was the ACT II trial.[11]

In this article, the authors discuss the existing evidence basis for the current treatment regimens. The authors review target delineation, optimized radiotherapy techniques, dose-escalation with external-beam radiotherapy (EBRT) or brachytherapy, and chemotherapy. The authors also speculate on novel approaches in terms of the integration of biological agents and immunotherapy, which are being developed for SCCA.

STRATEGIES FOR TREATING LOCALIZED ANAL CANAL CANCER
Radical Surgery

Up until the mid1980s, the standard treatment of SCCA involved surgery with a permanent colostomy. Local failure rates were reported between 27% and 47% and 5-year OS rates between 40% and 70% (depending on stage and extent of the disease at presentation). Although there has never been a randomized trial comparing radical surgery with radiotherapy or CRT, CRT achieves good local control without the inevitability of a permanent stoma.

Neoadjuvant/Induction Chemotherapy

NACT is widely used in cancers of the head and neck (SCC of the head and neck) before surgery or definitive CRT. In Europe a small pilot study treated SCCA with neoadjuvant 5-FU and cisplatin and showed an 82% response rate, with 27% achieving a complete clinical response (CCR).[20] A further study integrated neoadjuvant 5-FU/cisplatin[21] and showed CCR and partial response (PR) rates of 10% and 51% after NACT, 67% and 28% after CRT, and 93% and 5%, respectively, after all treatment was completed.

In the United States, the Cancer and Leukemia Group B (CALGB 9281) phase II study, for patients with larger, more advanced SCCA (cT3/T4) or with lymph node involvement (cN2/N3), evaluated induction chemotherapy using 5-FU (1000 mg/m^2 days 1–4 and 29–32) and cisplatin (100 mg/m^2 on days 1 and 29)[22] before CRT. The results showed 8 patients (18%) with CCR and 21 with PR in the 44 evaluable patients, and only a single patient had disease progression. After 4 years of follow-up, 27 of 44 (61%) were disease free.

Two randomized studies (RTOG 9811 and ACCORD-03) examined NACT based on the success of these results. Both incorporated split-course CRT. Additionally RTOG 9811 used 5-FU/cisplatin as the radio-sensitization for the CRT part of the treatment in place of MMC.[12,17] The results were virtually identical for the CALGB 9281 trial and the RTOG 9811 trial; but in the RTOG 9811 trial, only 26% of patients had tumors greater than 5 cm and positive nodes. Neither of the randomized trials documented the clinical response rates to NACT and whether responding patients had better locoregional control, disease-free survival, and OS.

It remains unclear from the reports of the RTOG 9811 trial whether total dose and/or planning target volumes were modified if patients achieved CCR or near CCR with NACT. There are no specific instructions in protocol. Hence, this may have introduced bias in the different arms, as the authors do not know whether the total dose of radiotherapy differed between induction and the MMC control arm. The studies also fail to report whether the gross target volume and clinical target volume were substantially different between arms or whether the pattern of relapse in the induction arm was different to the MMC control arm.

RADIOTHERAPY
External Beam Radiation Alone

EBRT was originally used as a single modality without chemotherapy. A control rate at the primary site of 75%[23] and OS rates at 5 years of 61% were reported. In a series of 270 patients,[24] local control was 90% for tumors less than 4 cm at 10 years but only 65% at 10 years for tumors greater than 4 cm. An early pooled analysis did not show a benefit for 5-FU/MMC in T1 tumors.[25] Some units, therefore, continue to treat small T1 tumors with radiation alone, although the ACT I trial suggested CRT is more effective, even for T1 tumors,[26] with a hazard ratio in favor of CRT similar to T2 and T3 cancers.

Retrospective studies suggest most recurrences occur locally at the primary site[1,2,6] often with involvement of adjacent structures and within the high-dose area.[1] Others have reported higher rates of regional recurrence when lower elective nodal doses are used, that is, inguinal failure (40%), common iliac (20%), external iliac (10%), internal iliac (10%), and presacral region (15%).[2] Nigro[6] reported that tumors greater than 4 cm in size were more difficult to control. Patients with lesions less than 3 cm in diameter and those treated strictly according to the protocol did significantly better than those with larger lesions and those whose treatment did not comply with the protocol.[27]

The optimal radiotherapy dose and fractionation for each clinical stage remains unknown. The data from the trials are muddied by limited information on the actual doses received, the overall treatment time (OTT), and the pattern of failure (local, locoregional, or distant). There are no data capturing the sites of locoregional failure in terms of the field size and target delineation, that is, within, marginal to, or outside of the prescribed dose for that radiotherapy field.

Preliminary data from the ACT II trial also suggest failure is usually in-field[4] and that locoregional failure in the elective nodal volume treated with 30.6 Gy was unusual, suggesting insufficient radiation dose or intrinsic radioresistance rather than inadequate clinical target volumes. Recently, a prospective phase II study evaluating intensity-modulated radiotherapy (IMRT) (RTOG O529)[28] suggested a reduction in acute toxicity compared with the RTOG 9811 trial using 2-dimensional and 3-dimensional techniques. IMRT may reduce the need for treatment breaks, which impact adversely on local control and allow dose-escalation in patients at high risk of local recurrence (T4N0 and T3-4N+). A national IMRT protocol for anal cancer has been developed in the UK (http://www.analimrtguidance.co.uk/analimrtguidance.pdf).

RADIOTHERAPY DOSE

In general, larger, more advanced cancers are more difficult to control than smaller ones and require higher doses of radiation, which in turn causes more morbidity. Identification of the optimal radiotherapy dose either with RT alone or CRT has been a challenge. Nigro[5] originally used a low dose of radiation, 30 Gy, in the CRT schedule as a preoperative neoadjuvant treatment before surgical resection. RTOG 8314[27] delivered 40.08 Gy in 4.5 to 5.0 weeks to the pelvis and perineum. Other prospective series increased the dose to 40 to 45 Gy delivered in 1.8 to 2.0 Gy per fraction[29] and achieved a complete response rate of 86%. Studies in older frail adults have also used lower doses for small tumors.[30,31]

Traditionally, a boost to the tumor with an interval after 45 Gy EBRT with or without chemotherapy has been used to achieve local control in high-risk patients. Most early trials used this schedule.[7-9] The ACCORD-03 trial, randomized eligible patients between standard (15 Gy) and higher boost doses (20–25 Gy), but also allowed the use of a higher radiotherapy boost dose if a poor clinical response was observed. The protocol allowed a 3-week gap between CRT and the boost, which will have diluted the effect of the higher dose. In addition, some trials introduced bias by allowing or even encouraging the investigator to boost with higher total doses if a lack of response in the primary was observed. The RTOG 9811 trial seems to recommend a minimum total dose of 45 Gy for good responders in T1/T2 cancers and higher doses for more advanced tumors or poor responders. The ACT II trial is the only trial that mandated a standard dose of 50.4 Gy to the primary tumor for all stages over 28 daily fractions using a 2-phase technique irrespective of response, with no gap between the phases.[11]

RTOG 9208 assessed an escalation of the radiotherapy dose to 59.6 Gy over 8.5 weeks with a mandatory 2-week gap. This schedule did not seem to improve local control but showed an increased 1- to 2-year colostomy rate compared with the RTOG 8704 outcomes whereby patients received a dose of only 45.0 to 50.4 Gy in 1.8 Gy per fraction.[32] A further 20 patient cohort was recruited with the same dose without treatment breaks, also showed no statistical significant difference in local relapse rate.[33]

Higher radiation doses using IMRT are proposed to improve these results, although there are concerns that the function of the sphincter mechanism will be compromised with greater than 54 to 56 Gy leading to fecal incontinence, poor function, and the eventual need for a defunctioning colostomy.[34] Long-term fecal incontinence in prostate cancer seems to correlate with the mean dose to the anal-sphincter region, with a cutoff when doses of greater than 40 Gy confer more risk.[35] Recent studies suggest that poor sphincter control correlates with doses of 53 Gy or greater received by the lateral extent of the anal sphincter region.[36]

Late complications of treatment represented 14.5% of the reasons for having a colostomy in the ACCORD-03 trial, that is, 9 of 307 (3%) of the overall population.[12] The RTOG 9811 trial reported severe long-term toxic effects in both arms of 11% and 10%, and 5% of patients required a colostomy for late effects.[10] In ACT II, 14 of 112 (12.5%) patients requiring a posttreatment colostomy needed this because of morbidity, that is, 14 of 940 (1.5%) overall.[37]

In general, adverse late effects reflect the total radiation dose rather than the type or dose of chemotherapy. With the exception of ACT II, total radiation doses have not been clearly documented in reports of the randomized trials. Sadly ACT II has not reported late toxicity, so a dose response model is, therefore, difficult to calculate.

ELECTIVE DOSE

The appropriate dose to elective nodal areas is also controversial. RTOG 8704 and RTOG 9811 prescribed doses of 30.6 Gy, 36 Gy, and 45 Gy to different areas of clinically negative nodes depending on their anatomic location. However, both the initial United Kingdom Coordinating Committee on Cancer Research (UKCCCR) and European Organization for Research and Treatment of Cancer (EORTC) trials used doses of 45 Gy to elective nodal stations. The RTOG 0529 prescribed 42 to 45 Gy to elective areas that appeared uninvolved on imaging and 50.4 Gy to inguino-pelvic lymph nodes less than 3 cm in size. Lymph nodes larger than 3 cm in size were treated to the same dose as the primary tumor, that is, 54 Gy. The elective nodal dose in ACT II was only 30.6 Gy in 17 daily fractions with large parallel, opposed fields.[11] Others have documented that CRT to elective nodal volumes (inguinal area and whole pelvis) over 4 weeks using a dose of 36 Gy achieved excellent nodal control.[38] Hence, a total of 30 Gy may be sufficient to treat microscopic nodal deposits and small-volume (<2 cm) macroscopic disease.

BRACHYTHERAPY

Brachytherapy is a highly conformal treatment that can deliver a high dose to the primary tumor, sparing surrounding normal tissues and the contralateral mucosa and sphincter. Implantation requires local or general anesthesia and demands skill and experience from the operator. Brachytherapy as a single modality is not recommended but may prove useful as a high-dose boost following response to CRT. Often a dose of 45 to 50 Gy using CRT is followed by a 15- to 20-Gy boost, delivered using interstitial brachytherapy. To avoid the risk of necrosis and/or treatment failure, the technique is probably best restricted to tumors that extend less than 50% of the circumference of the anal canal, are less than 5 to 10 mm in thickness, and are less than 5 cm in length.[39] Brachytherapy is a potentially useful technique both for the definitive and recurrent/salvage settings, but there is no consensus on the optimal fractionation schedule.[40] Double-plane or volume implants may be necessary, depending on the extent of the tumor. There is a risk of late necrosis and ongoing radiation proctitis. Recent reports of multiparametric MRI/computed tomography (CT) image adapted brachytherapy show the technique allows excellent dose distribution, but the expertise is limited.[41]

MAINTENANCE/CONSOLIDATION CHEMOTHERAPY FOLLOWING CHEMORADIATION

In SCCA a small retrospective study of advanced SCCA (61% were node positive and 43% T3/T4) suggested benefit for consolidation chemotherapy using 8 courses of chemotherapy with 5-FU/cisplatin following definitive CRT.[42] The ACT II trial in the United Kingdom randomly allocated 930 patients to 2 courses of maintenance/consolidation chemotherapy following CRT (5-FU 750 mg/m^2 for 4 days and cisplatin 60 mg/m^2 on day 1) versus control. This additional chemotherapy did not increase the CCR rate, the speed with which the tumor responded, or any long-term oncological outcomes, such as PFS or OS.[11,43]

THE OVERALL TREATMENT TIME

The interval between the different phases of radiation used in many trials may dilute the biological effects of a small boost of 5 to 10 Gy. Taking into account a repopulation constant with a presumed value of approximately 0.6 Gy/day[44] means only an additional 2.4 Gy may have been added by the boost in the ACT I trial, although with a 25-Gy boost this would have been closer to 12 Gy.[7] From these data and considering that local relapse remains the main site of failure, especially in locally advanced disease, a dose escalation might still be feasible and reasonable if IMRT is used and no planned gap is allowed, thus, optimizing the CRT component.

FIELD SIZE

Early trials used generous field sizes applied with parallel opposed beams to avoid a geometric miss, using the pelvic bones as reference points for the position of the pelvic nodes, based on data from lymphangiograms, CT scans and the histopathologic data from early radical surgical series.

Variations in field size exist between studies, particularly in the superior extent. Inclusion of the common iliac nodes, and full coverage of the entire internal iliac nodal system, by setting the upper CTV border at or above the sacral promontory[1,2] remains controversial. In ACT II the superior aspect of the initial anterior-posterior/posterior-anterior field was defined as 2 cm above the inferior aspect of the sacroiliac (SI) joints, usually at the S1/S2 interface; with beam divergence, the estimated dose to the common iliac nodes was small.[45] Very few isolated recurrences are observed above this field in the ACT II dataset.[4] In the RTOG's recommendations, common iliac nodes up to the fifth lumbar vertebra were included in the elective nodal volume to a dose of 45 Gy.[46,47] In the Norwegian National Population Cohort,[7] the recommended superior border was at the level of the lower border of the SI joints. Only if the primary cancer extended into rectal mucosa or the pelvic nodes were considered involved on imaging did the field extend up to the sacral promontory. Despite the fact that approximately 50% of patients had a field only extending to the lower end of the SI joint, no recurrences were observed above this treatment field. Hence, inclusion routinely of common iliac lymph nodes within the radiotherapy field may not be justified.

TARGET DELINEATION

CT planning relies on the contrast in tissue density between different organs. In SCCA, structures around the anal canal blend with indistinct organ borders. MRI can be coregistered to CT scans, offering better spatial resolution than either modality alone and defining tumor size, local extent and spread, invasion of adjacent organs, and nodal involvement.[48] Most anal carcinomas are also [18F] fluorodeoxyglucose avid, so metabolically active sites in both the primary tumor and normal-sized regional nodes can be identified with superior sensitivity compared with CT alone; but unlike MRI, images are not sharply delineated.

The RTOG, European Society for Radiotherapy and Oncology, and Australasian Gastro-Intestinal Trials Group have produced atlases for target delineation and prophylactic nodal irradiation[46,49] and also pelvic normal tissue contouring guidelines.[50] A recent UK initiative has also developed IMRT anal cancer guidance.[51]

RATIONALE FOR CHEMORADIOTHERAPY

The randomized trials in SCCA have only examined 3 cytotoxic agents as partners of radiotherapy (5-FU, MMC, and cisplatin). Although the schedules are similar (often days 1–5 and days 29–33), the doses, regimens, and OTT have not been consistent (**Table 2**). The strategy of continuous radio-sensitization throughout the radiotherapy currently accepted in rectal cancer (ie, prolonged venous infusion or oral capecitabine) has infrequently been exploited in anal cancer.[52,53]

Trials have never directly compared 1 or 2 doses of MMC, and so it remains unclear whether a second dose of MMC as used in some randomized trials[9,10] adds to efficacy. In Europe, several studies integrated concurrent cisplatin.[21,54,55] Various cisplatin doses have been explored in these different studies of CRT,[54,56,57] between 60 and 80 mg/m^2 on days 1 and 29, without an obvious advantage to the higher dose. An Eastern Cooperative Oncology Group (ECOG) phase II study (E4292) combined 2 courses of cisplatin 75 mg/m^2 on day 1 and 43 with a high dose of concurrent radiotherapy (59.4 Gy in 33 fractions), with a 2-week break after 36 Gy.[58] In total, 37% of patients experienced grade 4/5 toxicity. A second cohort received the same treatment without the planned treatment break and showed even more grade 4 toxicities.[59]

Cisplatin has only been explored in a weekly schedule in a single phase II study combined with MMC rather than 5-FU.[53] The EORTC 22011-40014 was initially planned as a randomized phase II/III trial designed to assess the response rate in the phase II component. The study compared 5-FU and MMC in combination with radiation versus MMC and cisplatin concurrent with radiation. The response rate of the MMC/cisplatin arm was 91.9%, satisfying the condition for phase III testing; but the investigators thought this regimen was not deliverable in a wider setting. Treatment with MMC has a lower median toxic dose (TD$_{50}$) and a more steeply increasing normal tissue complication probability curve compared with treatment with cisplatin.[60]

A combination of all 3 drugs in CRT (ie, 5-FU, MMC, and cisplatin) was investigated in a pilot study in the United Kingdom with a regimen using MMC at 10 mg/m^2 on day 1

Table 2
Outcomes of the more recent (1998–2008) phase III randomized trials in squamous cell carcinoma of the anus, the different chemoradiation regimens and outcomes

Studies (Authors)	Number of Patients	Median Follow-up	CCR	Local Failure Rate	DFS/RFS	Colostomy Rate/CFS	OS
RTOG 9811 (Ajani et al,[10] 2008)	644	2.5 y	No data on clinical response provided	25% with 5-FU, MMC vs 33% with 5-FU, cisplatin	DFS 60% with 5-FU, MMC vs 54% 5-FU, cisplatin at 5 y; NS P = .17	Colostomy rate: 10% with 5-FU, MMC vs 19% with 5-FU, cisplatin; P = .02 at 5 y	75% with 5-FU, MMC vs 70% with 5-FU, cisplatin; P = .1 at 5 y
ACCORD-03 (Peiffert et al,[12] 2012)	307	50 mo	Overall 79% complete clinical response at 2 mo after boost	Arm A 28% Arm B 12% Arm C 16% Arm D 22% Overall 19% at 5 y	Tumor-free survival Arm A 64% Arm B 78% Arm C 67% Arm D 62%	5-y CFS Arm A 70% Arm B 82% Arm C 77% Arm D 73%	5-y specific survival Arm A 77% Arm B 89% Arm C 81% Arm D 76%
UKCCCR ACT II (James et al,[11] 2013)	940	36 mo	94.5% 5-FU/MMC/RT vs 95% 5-FU/Cis/RT at 18 wk (ie, 12 wk before)	11% with MMC, 13% with cisplatin	RFS 75% in both arms at 3 y	Colostomy rate: same in both arms (5% with maintenance vs 4% without)	85% with maintenance at 3 y 84% without, NS

Abbreviations: Cis, Cisplatinum; HDRT, high-dose radiotherapy; NS, not significant; RFS, relapse-free survival; RT, radiotherapy.

and cisplatin 60 mg/m^2 on days 1 and 29,[61] but it was not taken forward because of concerns regarding acute toxicity and poor compliance.

ORAL FLUOROPYRIMIDINES

Capecitabine was successfully substituted for infusional 5-FU in a phase II study using 825 mg/m^2 twice a day on radiation days and MMC on day 1.[62] A more recent phase I study confirmed that 825 mg/m^2 twice a day orally is tolerable and seems effective.[63] Other phase II studies[64] and retrospective series[65,66] have confirmed this dosage as tolerable and effective (**Table 3**).

OTHER CYTOTOXIC AGENTS

A recent phase I trial of IMRT and concurrent chemotherapy using paclitaxel, capecitabine, and MMC for SCCA is reported in abstract. The regimen seems feasible in terms of toxicity, and 18 of 20 patients (90%) had a complete response at 6 months.[67] Based on these results, a phase III clinical trial is planned comparing the triplet regimen (paclitaxel, capecitabine, and MMC) combined with IMRT against the standard doublet of capecitabine and MMC alone (NCT02526953).

EPIDERMAL GROWTH FACTOR RECEPTOR INHIBITION

Epidermal growth factor receptor (EGFR) is overexpressed in up to 90% of SCCA. EGFR mutations, Kirsten rat sarcoma viral oncogene mutations, or BRAF mutations have rarely been identified in SCCA,[68,69] although one study showed PIK3CA was found to be mutated in 22%.[69] Thus, EGFR inhibition is a potential strategy to integrate

Table 3
Showing results of phase I/phase II and retrospective studies integrating capecitabine into chemoradiation regimens

Study	Number of Patients	Radiotherapy Dose	Schedule of MMC	Capecitabine	Local Control
Glynne-Jones et al,[62] 2008	31	50.4 Gy in 28 fractions in 2 phases	Single dose of MMC 12 mg/m^2 max 20 mg	825 mg/m^2 bid on radiation days	90% at 14 m
Deenen et al,[63] 2013	18	59.4 Gy in 33 fractions with simultaneous integrated boost-IMRT	Single dose of MMC 10 mg/m^2 max 15 mg	825 mg/m^2 bid on radiation days	88% at 28 m
Oliveira et al,[64] 2016	51	Not stated	Single dose of MMC 15 mg/m^2 on day 1	825 mg/m^2 bid on radiation days	86% at 6 m
Thind et al,[65] 2014	66	Median dose of radiation 51.9 Gy over 5.5 wk	Single dose of MMC 12 mg/m^2	825 mg/m^2 bid on radiation days	94% at 20 m
Wan et al,[66] 2014	300	50–54 Gy	Two doses But compliance poor if capecitabine	825 mg/m^2 bid on radiation days	DFS (at 1 y) 94% cape vs 91% 5-FU

into concurrent CRT treatment. In SCCA, several phase I studies investigated the addition of cetuximab to 5-FU and cisplatin-based CRT.[70] A response rate of 95% was observed, but the study closed early because of toxicity (52% showing severe grade 3–4 radiation dermatitis and 44% experiencing grade 3–4 diarrhea). The ACCORD 16 phase I trial also closed early because of unacceptable toxicity[71] and poor oncological outcomes.[72] Other phase II studies (ECOG 3205) for immunocompetent patients and (AIDS Malignancy Consortium Trial [AMC045]) human immunodeficiency virus (HIV)–positive patients showed acceptable toxicity and clinical outcomes for patients treated with the combination of cetuximab with 5-FU and cisplatin concurrently with radiation.[73] Other studies have combined cetuximab with 5-FU/MMC–based CRT.[75] Toxicity was acceptable, and 10 of 11 patients (91%) achieved a local complete remission (CR). A phase 2 trial with panitumumab, mitomycin-C, 5-FU, and radiotherapy in SCCA, has been developed by the Grupo Espanol Multidisciplinar en Cancer Digestivo (GEMCAD) - (NCT01285778).[76,77] Preliminary results showed only 55% had CR at 24 weeks (**Table 4**).

IMMUNOTHERAPY

Strong data support HPV infection as an early event in SCCA with reports of 84% to 85% HPV prevalence.[78,79] The two most common genotypes are HPV 16 and HPV 18. It is postulated that HPV integration at an early stage and loss of heterozygosity at multiple chromosomal sites may lead to anal carcinogenesis. Therefore, immunotherapy seems a promising approach and, as such, is being studied in combination with CRT.

Advaxis (ADXS) 11-001 is a bioengineered Listeria monocytogenes–based treatment combining live attenuated Listeria bacteria fused to HPV16E7 causing a cell-mediated immune response. ADXS 11-001 is being evaluated in a phase I/II study of 25 patients in combination with 5-FU and MMC and IMRT for anal cancer; this trial is currently recruiting (NCT01671488). ADXS 11-001 is also being tested with CRT in several other HPV-positive cancers, such as head and neck and cervical cancer.

The inhibitory molecules programmed cell death 1 (PD-1) and its ligands, PD-L1 and PD-L2, are often upregulated and lead to suppression of the antitumor immune response in many cancers. PDL1 expression has been associated with a worse prognosis; hence, checkpoint inhibition has proved successful in other tumor types. There is a paucity of data in SCCA, but one study of 41 patients evaluated PDL1 expression retrospectively using paraffin tissue blocks and identified 62% PDL1-positive in the late stage and 33% positive in the early stage. Although there were very small numbers, there was a suggestion of poorer relapse-free survival; but OS was not different between PDL1 positive and negative groups. Trials combining CRT with PDL1 blockade for anal cancer are currently being planned but will require cautious overview because of the potential overlapping gastrointestinal toxicities with CRT.

An evaluation of tumor-infiltrating lymphocytes (TIL) scores after chemoradiotherapy provides further support for immunotherapy in this setting.[80] P16 immunohistochemistry has been used as a surrogate for HPV involvement and demonstrated poor overall outcomes for HPV/p16-negative patients in several series.[81,82] One plausible explanation has been that the papillomavirus evokes a host immune response directed against tumor cells. In oropharyngeal cancer HPV 16–E6 and E7-specific T cells have been found and correlate with improved outcome. Thus, Gilbert and colleagues[80] assessed TIL to stratify p16-positive cases and demonstrated additional prognostic value with this approach. TILs remained an independent prognostic score in a multivariate analysis with relapse-free rates of 92% with high levels of TIL versus 63% in absent/low-level TIL.[80] These data support the use of immunotherapy either

Table 4
Showing preliminary and full results of phase I/phase II studies integrating cetuximab or panitumumab into chemoradiation regimens

Trial	No of Patients	IMRT	Regimen	Toxicity	Efficacy
Phase I Olivatto et al,[70] Cancer 2013	21 (stopped because of DLT)	No	5-FU/CP + RT + cetuximab	High	OK
Phase I ACCORD 16 Deutsch et al,[71] Ann Oncol 2013 Levy et al,[72] Radiother Oncol 2015	16 (stopped because of DLT)	No	5-FU/CP + RT + cetuximab	High	Low
Phase I Garg et al,[73] ECOG 3205, J Clin Oncol 2012 Garg et al,[74] J Clin Oncol 2016	28	Some	5-FU/CP + RT + cetuximab	G4 toxicity 32% G5 4%	93% OS at 2 y
Phase I Garg et al,[74] AMC045, J Clin Oncol 2016	45	Some	5-FU/CP + RT + cetuximab	G4 toxicity 26% G5 4%	89% OS at 2 y
Phase I Leon et al,[75] 2015	13	Yes	5-FU/MMC + RT + cetuximab	Low	73% CR at 3 mo
Phase II Feliu,[77] ASCO 2014	58 36 evaluable	No	5-FU/MMC + RT + panitumumab	High	At 24 wk 55% CR, 6% persistent disease; 19% progression

with concurrent CRT or using adoptive T-cell therapy that is being studied in trials in the advanced SCCA setting.

The Sonic hedgehog (SHH) glycoprotein is part of a complex signaling cascade that is regulated by Gli1. Ajani and colleagues[83] demonstrated that overexpression of Gli 1 and SHH glycoprotein were potentially predictive for reduced DFS.[83,84] These data support further interrogation of this pathway, especially as SHH signaling has been correlated with resistance to CRT in other cancers.

SUMMARY

Current guidelines from the European Society for Medical Oncology and the National Comprehensive Cancer Network recommend the use of concurrent CRT with 5-FU and MMC for radical treatment of local and locally advanced SCCA. Yet, we have not confirmed the optimal dose of radiotherapy or defined the schedules with the optimal sequence and timing of the available cytotoxic agents (5-FU, MMC, and cisplatin). Oral capecitabine offers an alternative to 5-FU but has not been directly compared with intravenous 5-FU in trials. Studies using the targeted agent cetuximab seem to cause unexpected toxicity, without showing any evidence of increased efficacy.

The response to chemoradiation is heterogeneous and may reflect the tumor environment and the immunologic capacity as much as innate radio-sensitivity. Biomarkers in development (p16, squamous cell carcinoma antigen, PET/CT, Tumor infiltrating lymphocytes, PD-1 expression, SHH expression) may stratify SCCA more accurately and guide the individual intensity of treatment required. In the future, we should integrate new agents, such as taxanes, checkpoint inhibitors, and PD-1, and molecularly targeted agents into CRT. The greater precision of IMRT can spare critical normal tissues, thereby reducing acute toxicity and potentially allowing the safe use of dose escalation. We also need to design trials specifically for patients with HPV-negative and HPV-positive SCCA both in smokers and nonsmokers, respectively, according to different TNM staging.

REFERENCES

1. Das P, Bhatia S, Eng C, et al. Predictors and patterns of recurrence after definitive chemoradiation for anal cancer. Int J Radiat Oncol Biol Phys 2007;68(3):794–800.
2. Wright JL, Patil S, Temple L, et al. Squamous cell carcinoma of the anal canal: patterns and predictors of failure and implications for intensity modulated radiation treatment planning. Int J Radiat Oncol Biol Phys 2009;78(4):1064–72.
3. Northover J, Glynne-Jones R, Sebag-Montefiore D, et al. Chemoradiation for the treatment of epidermoid anal cancer: 13-year follow-up of the first randomised UKCCCR Anal Cancer Trial (ACT I). Br J Cancer 2010;102(7):1123–8.
4. Sebag-Montefiore D, James R, Meadows H, et al. The pattern and timing of disease recurrence in squamous cancer of the anus: mature results from the NCRI ACT II trial. J Clin Oncol 2012;30(Suppl) [abstract: 4029].
5. Nigro ND, Vaitkevicius VK, Considine B Jr. Combined therapy for cancer of the anal canal: a preliminary report. Dis Colon Rectum 1974;17(3):354–6.
6. Nigro ND. An evaluation of combined therapy for squamous call carcinoma of the anal canal. Dis Colon Rectum 1984;27:763–6.
7. UKCCCR Anal Cancer Working Party. Epidermoid Anal Cancer: results from the UKCCCR randomised trial of radiotherapy alone versus radiotherapy, 5-fluorouracil and mitomycin. Lancet 1996;348:1049–54.
8. Bartelink H, Roelofsen F, Eschwege F, et al. Concomitant radiotherapy and chemotherapy is superior to radiotherapy alone in the treatment of locally

advanced anal cancer: results of a phase III randomized trial of the European Organization for Research and Treatment of Cancer Radiotherapy and Gastrointestinal Cooperative Groups. J Clin Oncol 1997;15(5):2040–9.

9. Flam M, John M, Pajak TF, et al. Role of mitomycin in combination with fluorouracil and radiotherapy, and of salvage chemoradiation in the definitive nonsurgical treatment of epidermoid carcinoma of the anal canal: results of a phase III randomized intergroup study. J Clin Oncol 1996;14(9):2527–39.

10. Ajani JA, Winter KA, Gunderson LL, et al. Fluorouracil, mitomycin, and radiotherapy vs fluorouracil, cisplatin, and radiotherapy for carcinoma of the anal canal: a randomized controlled trial. JAMA 2008;299(16):1914–21.

11. James RD, Glynne-Jones R, Meadows H, et al. Mitomycin or cisplatin chemoradiation with or without maintenance chemotherapy for treatment of squamous-cell carcinoma of the anus (ACT II): a randomised, phase 3, open-label, 2x2 factorial trial. Lancet Oncol 2013;14:516–24.

12. Peiffert D, Tournier-Rangeard L, Gerard JP, et al. Induction chemotherapy and dose intensification of the radiation boost in locally advanced anal canal carcinoma: final analysis of the randomized UNICANCER ACCORD 03 trial. J Clin Oncol 2012;30:1941–4.

13. Glynne-Jones R, Nilsson PJ, Aschele C, et al. Anal cancer: ESMO-ESSO-ESTRO clinical practice guidelines for diagnosis treatment and follow up. Ann Oncol 2014;25(Suppl 3):iii10–20.

14. NCCN. NCCN Clinical Practice Guidelines in Oncology: anal carcinoma, version 2, 2016. Available at: https://www.nccn.org/professionals/physician_gls/f_guidelines.asp. Accessed August 12, 2016.

15. Gunderson LL, Winter KA, Ajani JA, et al. Long-term update of U.S. GI Intergroup RTOG 98-11 phase III trial for anal carcinoma: survival, relapse and colostomy failure with concurrent chemoradiation involving fluorouracil/mitomycin versus fluorouracil/cisplatin. J Clin Oncol 2012;30:4344–51.

16. Bentzen AG, Guren MG, Vonen B, et al. Faecal incontinence after chemoradiotherapy in anal cancer survivors: long-term results of a national cohort. Radiother Oncol 2013;108(1):55–60.

17. Gunderson LL, Moughan J, Ajani JA, et al. Anal carcinoma: impact of TN category of disease on survival, disease relapse, and colostomy failure in US Gastrointestinal Intergroup RTOG 98-11 phase 3 trial. Int J Radiat Oncol Biol Phys 2013;87(4):638–45.

18. Withers HR, Taylor JMF, Maciejewski B. The hazard of accelerated tumour clonage and repopulation during radiotherapy. Acta Oncol 1988;27:131–46.

19. Fowler JF, Lindstrom MJ. Loss of local control with prolongation in radiotherapy. Int J Radiat Oncol Biol Phys 1992;23:457–67.

20. Brunet R, Sadek H, Vignoud J, et al. Cisplatin (P) and 5 fluorouracil (5FU), for the neoadjuvant treatment (Tt) of epidermoid anal canal carcinoma (EACC) [abstract]. Proc Am Soc Clin Oncol 1990;9:104.

21. Peiffert D, Giovannini M, Ducreux M, et al. Digestive Tumours Group of the French 'Fédération Nationale des Centres de Lutte Contre le Cancer'. High-dose radiation therapy and neoadjuvant plus concomitant chemotherapy with 5-fluorouracil and cisplatin in patients with locally advanced squamous-cell anal canal cancer: final results of a phase II study. Ann Oncol 2001;12(3):397–404.

22. Meropol NJ, Niedzwiecki D, Shank B, et al. Induction therapy for poor-prognosis anal canal carcinoma: a phase II study of the cancer and leukemia group B (CALGB 9281). J Clin Oncol 2008;26(19):3229–34.

23. Ng Ying Kin NY, Pigneux J, Auvray H, et al. Our experience of conservative treatment of anal canal carcinoma combining external irradiation and interstitial implant: 32 cases treated between 1973 and 1982. Int J Radiat Oncol Biol Phys 1988;14(2):253–9.

24. Touboul E, Schlienger M, Buffat L, et al. Epidermoid carcinoma of the anal canal. Results of curative-intent radiation therapy in a series of 270 patients. Cancer 1994;73(6):1569–79.

25. Cummings BJ, Keane TJ, O'Sullivan B, et al. Epidermoid anal cancer: treatment by radiation alone or by radiation and 5-fluorouracil with and without mitomycin C. Int J Radiat Oncol Biol Phys 1991;21(5):1115–25.

26. Northover J, Meadows H, Ryan C, et al. Combined radiotherapy and chemotherapy for anal cancer. The Lancet 1997;349:205–6.

27. Sischy B, Doggett RL, Krall JM, et al. Definitive irradiation and chemotherapy for radiosensitization in management of anal carcinoma: interim report on Radiation Therapy Oncology Group Study No. 8314. J Natl Cancer Inst 1989;81:850–6.

28. Kachnic LA, Winter K, Myerson RJ, et al. RTOG 0529: a phase 2 evaluation of dose-painted intensity modulated radiation therapy in combination with 5-fluorouracil and mitomycin-C for the reduction of acute morbidity in carcinoma of the anal canal. Int J Radiat Oncol Biol Phys 2013;86(1):27–33.

29. Flam MS, John MJ, Mowry PA, et al. Definitive combined modality therapy of carcinoma of the anus. A report of 30 cases including results of salvage therapy in patients with residual disease. Dis Colon Rectum 1987;30(7):495–502.

30. Hu K, Minsky BD, Cohen AM, et al. 30 Gy may be an adequate dose in patients with anal cancer treated with excisional biopsy followed by combined-modality therapy. J Surg Oncol 1999;70:71–7.

31. Hatfield P, Cooper R, Sebag-Montefiore D. Involved-field, low-dose chemoradiotherapy for early-stage anal carcinoma. Int J Radiat Oncol Biol Phys 2008;70:419–24.

32. John M, Pajak T, Flam M, et al. Dose escalation in chemoradiation for anal cancer: preliminary results of RTOG 92-08. Cancer J Sci Am 1996;2:205–11.

33. Konski A, Garcia M Jr, John M, et al. Evaluation of planned treatment breaks during radiation therapy for anal cancer: update of RTOG 92-08. Int J Radiat Oncol Biol Phys 2008;72:114–8.

34. Broens P, Van Limbergen E, Penninckx F, et al. Clinical and manometric effects of combined external beam irradiation and brachytherapy for anal cancer. Int J Colorectal Dis 1998;13:68–72.

35. Alsadius D, Hedelin M, Lundstedt D, et al. Mean absorbed dose to the anal-sphincter region and fecal leakage among irradiated prostate cancer survivors. Int J Radiat Oncol Biol Phys 2012;84(2):e181–5.

36. Buettner F, Gulliford SL, Webb S, et al. The dose-response of the anal sphincter region–an analysis of data from the MRC RT01 trial. Radiother Oncol 2012;103(3):347–52.

37. Glynne-Jones R, Kadalayil L, Meadows HM, et al, on behalf of ACT II Study Group. Tumour- and treatment-related colostomy rates following mitomycin C or cisplatin chemoradiation with or without maintenance chemotherapy in squamous cell carcinoma of the anus in the ACT II trial. Ann Oncol 2014;25(8):1616–22.

38. Lepinoy A, Lescut N, Puyraveau M, et al. Evaluation of a 36Gy elective node irradiation dose in anal cancer. Radiother Oncol 2015;116(2):197–201.

39. Mazeron JJ, van Limbergen E. Anorectal cancer. In: Gerbaulet A, Pötter R, Mazeron J, et al, editors. The GECESTROH and book of brachy therapy. Brussels (Belgium): ESTRO; 2000. p. 505–14.

40. Niehoff P, Kovacs G. HDR brachytherapy for anal cancer. J Gastrointest Oncol 2014;5(3):218–22.

41. Tagliaferri L, Manfrida S, Barbaro B, et al. MITHRA – multiparametric MR/CT image adapted brachytherapy (MR/CT-IABT) in anal canal cancer: a feasibility study. J Contemp Brachytherapy 2015;7(5):336–45.
42. Glynne-Jones R, James R, Meadows H, et al. Optimum time to assess complete clinical response (CR) following chemoradiation (CRT) using mitomycin (MMC) or cisplatin (CisP), with or without maintenance CisP/5FU in squamous cell carcinoma of the anus: results of ACT II. J Clin Oncol 2012;30(Suppl) [abstract: 4004].
43. Cho BC, Ahn JB, Seong J, et al. Chemoradiotherapy with or without consolidation chemotherapy using cisplatin and 5-fluorouracil in anal squamous cell carcinoma: long-term results in 31 patients. BMC Cancer 2008;15:8.
44. Glynne-Jones R, Sebag-Montefiore D, Adams R, et al. "Mind the gap"–the impact of variations in the duration of the treatment gap and overall treatment time in the first UK Anal Cancer Trial (ACT I). Int J Radiat Oncol Biol Phys 2011;81(5): 1488–94.
45. Aggarwal A, Gayadeen S, Robinson D, et al. Clinical target volumes in anal cancer: calculating what dose was likely to have been delivered in the UK ACT II trial protocol. Radiother Oncol 2012;103(3):341–6.
46. Myerson RJ, Garofalo MC, Naqa I, et al. Elective clinical target volumes for conformal therapy in anorectal cancer: a radiation therapy oncology group consensus panel contouring atlas. Int J Radiat Oncol Biol Phys 2009;74(3): 824–30.
47. Bentzen AG, Guren MG, Wanderås EH, et al. Chemoradiotherapy of anal carcinoma: survival and recurrence in an unselected national cohort. Int J Radiat Oncol Biol Phys 2012;83(2):e173–80.
48. Goh V, Gollub FK, Liaw J, et al. Magnetic resonance imaging assessment of squamous cell carcinoma of the anal canal before and after chemoradiation: can MRI predict for eventual clinical outcome? Int J Radiat Oncol Biol Phys 2010;78(3):715–21.
49. Ng M, Leong T, Chander S, et al. Australasian Gastrointestinal Trials Group (AGITG) contouring atlas and planning guidelines for intensity-modulated radiotherapy in anal cancer. Int J Radiat Oncol Biol Phys 2012;83:1455–62.
50. Gay HA, Barthold HJ, O'Meara E, et al. Pelvic normal tissue contouring guidelines for radiation therapy: a Radiation Therapy Oncology Group consensus panel atlas. Int J Radiat Oncol Biol Phys 2012;83:e353–62.
51. Muirhead R, Adams RA, Gilbert DC, et al. Anal cancer: developing an intensity-modulated radiotherapy solution for ACT2 fractionation. Clin Oncol (R Coll Radiol) 2014;26:720–1.
52. Bosset JF, Roelofsen F, Morgan DA, et al. Shortened irradiation scheme, continuous infusion of 5-fluorouracil and fractionation of mitomycin C in locally advanced anal carcinomas. Results of a phase II study of the European Organization for Research and Treatment of Cancer. Radiotherapy and Gastrointestinal Cooperative Groups. Eur J Cancer 2003;39(1):45–51.
53. Matzinger O, Roelofsen F, Mineur L, et al. Mitomycin C with continuous fluorouracil or with cisplatin in combination with radiotherapy for locally advanced anal cancer (European Organisation for Research and Treatment of Cancer phase II study 22011-40014). Eur J Cancer 2009;45(16):2782–91.
54. Doci R, Zucali R, Bombelli L, et al. Combined chemoradiation therapy for anal cancer. A report of 56 cases. Ann Surg 1992;215(2):150–6.
55. Gerard JP, Ayzac L, Hun D, et al. Treatment of anal canal carcinoma with high dose radiation therapy and concomitant fluorouracil-cisplatinum. Long-term results in 95 patients. Radiother Oncol 1998;46(3):249–56.

56. Hung A, Crane C, Delclos M, et al. Cisplatin-based combined modality therapy for anal carcinoma: a wider therapeutic index. Cancer 2003;97(5):1195–202.

57. Olivatto LO, Cabral V, Rosa A, et al. Mitomycin-C- or cisplatin-based chemoradio-therapy for anal canal carcinoma: long-term results. Int J Radiat Oncol Biol Phys 2011;79(2):490–5.

58. Martenson JA, Lipsitz SR, Wagner H Jr, et al. Initial results of a phase II trial of high dose radiation therapy, 5-fluorouracil, and cisplatin for patients with anal cancer (E4292): an Eastern Cooperative Oncology Group study. Int J Radiat On-col Biol Phys 1996;35(4):745–9.

59. Chakravarthy AB, Catalano PJ, Martenson JA, et al. Long-term follow-up of a phase II trial of high-dose radiation with concurrent 5-fluorouracil and cisplatin in patients with anal cancer (ECOG E4292). Int J Radiat Oncol Biol Phys 2011; 81(4):e607–13.

60. Bazan JG, Luxton G, Kozak MM, et al. Impact of chemotherapy on normal tissue complication probability models of acute hematologic toxicity in patients receiving pelvic intensity modulated radiation therapy. Int J Radiat Oncol Biol Phys 2013;87(5):983–91.

61. Sebag-Montefiore D, Meadows HM, Cunningham D, et al. Three cytotoxic drugs combined with pelvic radiation and as maintenance chemotherapy for patients with squamous cell carcinoma of the anus (SCCA): long-term follow-up of a phase II pilot study using 5-fluorouracil, mitomycin C and cisplatin. Radiother On-col 2012;104(2):155–60.

62. Glynne-Jones R, Meadows H, Wan S, et al. EXTRA–a multicenter phase II study of chemoradiation using a 5 day per week oral regimen of capecitabine and intrave-nous mitomycin C in anal cancer. Int J Radiat Oncol Biol Phys 2008;72(1):119–26.

63. Deenen MJ, Dewit L, Boot H, et al. Simultaneous integrated boost-intensity modu-lated radiation therapy with concomitant capecitabine and mitomycin C for locally advanced anal carcinoma: a phase 1 study. Int J Radiat Oncol Biol Phys 2013; 85(5):e201–7.

64. Oliveira SC, Moniz CM, Riechelmann R, et al. Phase II study of capecitabine in substitution of 5-FU in the chemoradiotherapy regimen for patients with localized squamous cell carcinoma of the anal canal. J Gastrointest Cancer 2016;47(1): 75–81.

65. Thind G, Johal B, Follwell M, et al. Chemoradiation with capecitabine and mitomycin-C for stage I-III anal squamous cell carcinoma. Radiat Oncol 2014; 9:124.

66. Wan DDC, Schellenberg D, Hay J, et al. A comparison between 5-fluorouracil/ mitomycin (FM) and capecitabine/mitomycin (CM) in combination with radiation (RT) for squamous cell carcinoma (SCC) of the anal canal. J Clin Oncol 2014; 32(5s) [abstract: 4031].

67. Gordeev S, Rasulov A, Gorbunova V, et al. A pilot study of intensity-modulated radiation therapy (IMRT) and concurrent chemotherapy (CT) with paclitaxel, ca-pecitabine and mitomycin C for squamous cell anal carcinoma (SCAC). J Clin Oncol 2015;33(Suppl) [abstract: e14501].

68. Casadei Gardini A, Capelli L, Ulivi P, et al. KRAS, BRAF and PIK3CA status in squamous cell anal carcinoma (SCAC). PLoS One 2014;9(3):e92071.

69. Serup-Hansen E, Linnemann D, Høgdall E, et al. KRAS and BRAF mutations in anal carcinoma. APMIS 2015;123(1):53–9.

70. Olivatto LO, Vieira FM, Pereira BV, et al. Phase 1 study of cetuximab in combina-tion with 5-fluorouracil, cisplatin, and radiotherapy in patients with locally advanced anal canal carcinoma. Cancer 2013;119(16):2973–80.

71. Deutsch E, Lemanski C, Pignon JP, et al. Unexpected toxicity of cetuximab combined with conventional chemoradiotherapy in patients with locally advanced anal cancer: results of the UNICANCER ACCORD 16 phase II trial. Ann Oncol 2013;24:2834–8.
72. Levy A, Azria D, Pignon JP, et al. Low response rate after cetuximab combined with conventional chemoradiotherapy in patients with locally advanced anal cancer: long-term results of the UNICANCER ACCORD 16 phase II trial. Radiother Oncol 2015;114(3):415–6.
73. Garg M, Lee JY, Kachnic LA, et al. Phase II trials of cetuximab (CX) plus cisplatin (CDDP), 5fluorouracil (5-FU) and radiation (RT) in immunocompetent (ECOG 3205) and HIV-positive (AMC045) patients with squamous cell carcinoma of the anal canal (SCAC): safety and preliminary efficacy results. J Clin Oncol ASCO Annual Meeting Proceedings. 2012. [abstract: 4030].
74. Garg M, Lee JY, Lisa A, et al. Phase II trials of cetuximab (CX) plus cisplatin (CDDP), 5-fluorouracil (5-FU) and radiation (RT) in immunocompetent (ECOG 3205) and HIV-positive (AMC045) patients with squamous cell carcinoma of the anal canal (SCAC): Safety and preliminary efficacy results. J Clin Oncol 34, 2016 (suppl; abstr 3522).
75. Leon O, Guren MG, Radu C, et al. Phase I study of cetuximab in combination with 5-fluorouracil, mitomycin C and radiotherapy in patients with locally advanced anal cancer. Eur J Cancer 2015;51(18):2740–6.
76. Moreno V, García-Carbonero R, Maurel J, et al. Phase 1 study of cetuximab in combination with 5-fluorouracil, cisplatin, and radiotherapy in patients with locally advanced anal canal carcinoma. Cancer 2014;120(3):454–6.
77. Feliu J, Garcia-Carbonero R, Capdevila J, et al. Phase II trial of panitumumab (P) plus mitomycin C (M), 5-fluorouracil (5-FU), and radiation (RT) in patients with squamous cell carcinoma of the anal canal (SCAC): safety and efficacy profile—VITAL study, GEMCAD 09-02 clinical trial. J Clin Oncol 2014;32(5s) [abstract: 4034].
78. Hoots BE, Palefsky JM, Pimenta JM, et al. Human papilloma virus type distribution in anal cancer and anal intraepithelial lesions. Int J Cancer 2009;124:2375–83.
79. Palmer JG, Scholefield JH, Coates PJ, et al. Anal cancer and human papilloma viruses. Dis Colon Rectum 1989;32:16–22.
80. Gilbert DC, Serup–Hansen E, Linnemann D, et al. Tumour infiltrating lymphocytes scores effectively stratify outcomes over and above p16 post chemoradiotherapy in anal cancer. Br J Cancer 2016;114:134–7.
81. Koerber SA, Schoneweg C, Slynko A, et al. Influence of human papillomavirus and p16 on treatment outcome of patients with anal cancer. Radiother Oncol 2014;113:331–6.
82. Rodel F, Wieland U, Fraunholz I, et al. Human papilloma virus DNA load and p16INK4a expression predict for local control in patients with anal squamous carcinoma treated with chemoradiotherapy. Int J Cancer 2014;136:278–88.
83. Ajani JA, Wang X, Izzo JG, et al. Molecular biomarkers correlate with disease free survival in patients with anal cell carcinoma treated with chemoradiation. Dig Dis Sci 2010;55:1098–105.
84. Sims-Mourtada J, Izzo JG, Apisarnthanarax S, et al. Hedgehog: an attribute to tumour regrowth after chemoradiotherapy and a target to improve radiation response. Clin Cancer Res 2006;12:6565–72.

Evolution and Management of Treatment-Related Toxicity in Anal Cancer

 CrossMark

Ethan B. Ludmir, MD[a], Lisa A. Kachnic, MD[b], Brian G. Czito, MD[c],*

KEYWORDS

- Anal cancer • Chemoradiation • Radiotherapy • Chemotherapy • Toxicity
- Intensity-modulated radiotherapy • Mitomycin-C • Cisplatin

KEY POINTS

- Definitive chemoradiation (CRT) regimens in the treatment of anal cancer have evolved over successive clinical trials.
- Although cure rates are high with these regimens, they result in hematologic, dermatologic, gastrointestinal (GI), and genitourinary (GU) toxicities.
- Alternative strategies, including novel radiotherapy approaches as well as novel chemotherapeutics, are aimed at reducing treatment-related toxicity without having a negative impact on disease-related outcomes.
- Toxicity management often requires algorithmic and multidisciplinary approaches; contemporary studies are focusing on long-term quality-of-life sequelae following anal cancer treatment.

INTRODUCTION

Anal cancer is an uncommon malignancy whose incidence has been rising over the past several decades.[1] In 2016, it is expected that more than 8000 new cases of anal cancer will be diagnosed in the United States, resulting in more than 1000 deaths.[2] Since the 1970s, curative treatment of nonmetastatic anal cancer has increasingly centered on definitive RT, which now is established as the primary treatment. Although anal cancer is largely curable with CRT, these treatments are associated with a substantial toxicity profile. Many of the large randomized clinical trials (RCTs) for anal cancer have focused on mitigating toxicity without compromising

The authors have nothing to disclose.
[a] Department of Radiation Oncology, The University of Texas MD Anderson Cancer Center, 1400 Pressler St, Unit 1422, Houston, TX 77030, USA; [b] Department of Radiation Oncology, Vanderbilt University Medical Center, 2220 Pierce Avenue, Suite B1034, Nashville, TN 37232, USA; [c] Department of Radiation Oncology, Duke University Medical Center, Box 3085, Durham, NC 27710, USA
* Corresponding author.
E-mail address: czito001@mc.duke.edu

outcomes. This review focuses on the evolution of treatment-related toxicity for anal cancer with the progression of RCTs over the past several decades. As the standard of care has changed with the results of these RCTs, so too has the toxicity profile for anal cancer treatment. Management of these adverse effects is reviewed as are future directions in the treatment of anal cancer and their impact on toxicity.

TOXICITY DURING THE SURGICAL ERA

Prior to the advent and acceptance of definitive nonsurgical treatment options for anal carcinoma, abdominoperineal resection (APR) represented the standard of care. From an outcomes perspective, definitive APR alone resulted in recurrence rates of approximately 40% in patients treated with curative-intent.[3] Similarly, 5-year overall survival (OS) rates with APR alone averaged 62%, ranging between 51% and 71% in most studies.[3–5] In addition to these limitations, APR entails significant morbidity: as a non–sphincter-preserving procedure (ie, the entire anal sphincter complex is removed), permanent colostomy rate is 100%, along with high rates of urinary/sexual dysfunction, wound morbidity, and additional perioperative morbidity and mortality.

With this in mind, Nigro and colleagues[6] at Wayne State University piloted an effort in the early 1970s to assess the role of neoadjuvant CRT, combining 30 Gy to 35 Gy external-beam radiotherapy (EBRT) with concurrent 5-fluorouracil (5-FU) and mitomycin-C (MMC). In their initial report, these investigators demonstrated pathologic complete response (CR) in 2 patients treated with neoadjuvant CRT followed by APR.[6] The possibility of definitive CRT obviating subsequent APR resulted in the expansion of their efforts, culminating in a report of 45 patients treated with 30 Gy EBRT plus concurrent 5-FU/MMC. Remarkably, post-CRT biopsy specimens demonstrated CR in 84% of patients, with no subsequent recurrence in those with biopsy-proven CR. Of these 45 patients, 11% experienced grade 3 or higher hematologic toxicity. The investigators also reported "low-grade stomatitis" and "moderate diarrhea" as part of the acute toxicity profile of their regimen.[7,8] With these promising results, definitive surgical management of anal carcinoma ultimately gave way to definitive CRT; subsequent RCTs have therefore focused on the optimal nonsurgical approach for anal cancer.

In the modern era, the role of definitive surgical treatment of previously untreated anal lesions is primarily in the setting of T1N0 well-differentiated anal margin cancer.[9,10] These lesions, with highly favorable prognoses, may be treated with wide local excision; radiotherapy (RT) (with or without concurrent chemotherapy) is reserved for cases where re-excision (for positive or close margins) is not possible.[9,10] Given this limited scope for definitive surgery, the remainder of this review focuses on the toxicities associated with definitive CRT regimens for these patients.

FIRST-GENERATION TRIALS—RADIOTHERAPY VERSUS CHEMORADIOTHERAPY

Concurrent with the Nigro protocol, other experiences suggested that RT alone could also achieve promising outcomes.[11] Similarly, the toxicities associated with the Nigro chemotherapeutics (in particular MMC) further spurred the question as to whether RT could be as efficacious as CRT but with fewer adverse effects. Two RCTs were conducted to assess outcomes and toxicity profiles with RT versus CRT as definitive treatment of anal cancer: the United Kingdom Coordinating Committee on Cancer Research (UKCCCR) Anal Cancer Trial (ACT I), and the European Organisation for Research and Treatment of Cancer (EORTC) trial.[12–14] Both ACT I and EORTC trials used a 45 Gy RT regimen and prescribed similar concurrent 5-FU/MCC chemotherapy regimens for the CRT arms. Both trials involved a 6-week post-treatment break and additional boost RT to partial and complete responders; definitive surgery after the 6-week break was pursued for nonresponding patients. Both the ACT I and EORTC trials demonstrated improved locoregional control (LRC) as well as decreased colostomy rates with CRT (**Table 1**). At 5 years, the LRC rates for the CRT arm versus the RT arm were 68% versus 43% in ACT I and 68% versus 51% in EORTC, with corresponding 5-year colostomy-free survival (CFS) rates of 47% versus 37% and 72% versus 40%, respectively.[13,14] In long-term follow-up of the ACT I trial, it was further demonstrated that risk of death due to anal cancer was significantly decreased in the CRT group.[13]

With these results, ACT I and EORTC established CRT with 5-FU/MMC as the standard of care for definitive treatment of anal cancer. However, the outcomes benefits observed with the addition of 5-FU/MMC came with the sequelae of increased treatment-related toxicities, primarily skin, GU, GI , and hematologic toxicities (see **Table 1**). In ACT I, which enrolled more than 5-fold the number of patients as the EORTC trial, total early morbidity was significantly higher for the CRT arm (48% vs 39%).[12] **Table 1** provides a breakdown of these toxicities. Notably, hematologic toxicity was exclusively observed in the CRT arm. As later studies would confirm, MMC is the primary driver of these acute hematologic effects. ACT I investigators reported 6 chemotherapy-related deaths in the CRT arm (N = 292), 2 of which occurred within 18 months of treatment. These deaths resulted in dose-reduction protocol changes for the frail and elderly. Also reported in ACT I were 3 RT-related deaths (1 in the RT arm [N = 285] and 2 in the CRT arm [N = 292]). With far smaller sample sizes, the EORTC trial reported nonsignificant but higher rates of severe skin reactions and diarrhea in the CRT arm.[14] The sole treatment death in EORTC was in the CRT arm (N = 51), due to neutropenic sepsis during treatment.

Whereas acute toxicities were generally more prominent in the CRT arms of both trials, the late toxicities were similar across treatment groups. In both the initial ACT I and the 13-year long-term follow-up reports, late morbidity was similar between CRT and RT arms, including cutaneous, GU, and GI toxicities (see **Table 1**).[12,13] The EORTC data echoed these findings, with the exception of a higher rate of anal ulcer development in the CRT arm (18% vs 4%).[14] The EORTC trial also demonstrated no difference in the severe toxicity-free interval survival between the 2 arms. Collectively, these first-generation trials demonstrated superior disease-related outcomes, including CFS, for CRT versus RT, at the expense of increased acute toxicity.

SECOND-GENERATION TRIALS—MITOMYCIN AND CISPLATIN
Role of Mitomycin—RTOG 87-04

With the establishment of definitive CRT as standard of care, the component parts of the 5-FU/MMC regimen fell under scrutiny. Given the significant toxicity profile of MMC (thrombocytopenia, leukopenia, pulmonary toxicity, nephrotoxicity, and hemolytic-uremic syndrome), smaller trials had attempted to address the efficacy of 5-FU/RT regimens with and without MMC.[15–17] These efforts culminated in the Radiation Therapy Oncology Group (RTOG) 87-04 trial.[18] This study randomized patients to 5-FU/RT regimens with or without concurrent MMC. Although the RT (45 Gy) and 5-FU regimens were comparable to the ACT I and EORTC trials, the American RTOG 87-04 trial differed from its European counterparts in that MMC was dosed twice—10 mg/m^2 on days 1 and 29 (vs a single dose of 12 mg/m^2 or 15 mg/m^2 on day 1 in the ACT I and EORTC trials, respectively).[12,14,18] These differences in MMC dosing between trials, and their potential impact on outcomes and toxicities, are discussed later. At 4-year follow-up, improved disease-related outcomes with the

Table 1
First-generation trial outcomes and toxicity profiles

Trial	Comparison	Disease-Related Outcomes			Acute Toxicities				Late Toxicities			
		Locoregional Control	Overall Survival	Colostomy-free Survival	Hematologic	Skin	Gastrointestinal	Genitourinary	Skin	Gastrointestinal	Genitourinary	Other
ACT I (Arnott et al,[12] 1996; Northover et al,[13] 2010)	RT + 5-FU/MMC vs RT-alone	68% vs 43%, 5 y	58% vs 53%, 5 y	47% vs 37%, 5 y	Leukopenia: 7% vs 0%; Thrombocytopenia: 5% vs 0%	Severe skin toxicity: 17% vs 14%	Severe GI toxicity: 5% vs 2%	Severe GU toxicity: 1% vs 0%	21% vs 18%	Anorectal: 29% vs 27%	4% vs 4%	Ulcers/radionecrosis: 8% vs 6%
EORTC (Bartelink et al,[14] 1997)	RT + 5-FU/MMC vs RT-alone	68% vs 51%, 5 y	58% vs 53%, 5y	72% vs 40%, 5y	NR	Grade 3–4 skin reaction: 60% vs 50%	Grade 3–4 diarrhea: 20% vs 8%	NR	Skin ulceration: 6% vs 4%; severe fibrosis: 6% vs 8%	Anal ulcer: 18% vs 4%; anal fistula: 4% vs 6%; anal perforation: 4% vs 4%; rectal stenosis: 6% vs 4%	NR	NR

Abbreviation: NR, not reported.

addition of MMC were seen. As shown in **Table 2**, the addition of MMC significantly improved CFS (71% vs 59%), local control (84% vs 66%), and disease-free survival (DFS) (73% vs 51%).[18] Although not statistically significant, 4-year OS was also higher in the MMC group (76% vs 67%). These benefits, however, came at the expense of primarily hematologic MMC-related toxicities. Total acute toxicity rate, defined as grade 4 to 5 toxicities experienced within 90 days of treatment initiation, were significantly higher in the MMC arm (20% vs 7%). Stratifying these acute adverse effects, similar nonhematologic toxicities were observed between the arms (7% vs 4%), with hematologic toxicities significantly higher with the addition of MMC (18% vs 3%) (see **Table 2**). The severity of the neutropenia associated with MMC was reflected in the treatment-related deaths as well. Five treatment-related deaths, all due to neutropenic sepsis, were reported: 4 in the MMC arm (N = 146) and 1 in the non-MMC arm (N = 145). Late toxicities were similar between the 2 arms (5% vs 1%) (see **Table 2**). Despite the hematologic effects of MMC, the significant improvement in disease-related outcomes further supported RT + 5-FU/MMC as the standard of care.

Roles of Cisplatin and Induction Therapy—RTOG 98-11, ACCORD 03, and ACT II

Concurrent with RTOG 87-04, phase II trials sought to determine if an alternative chemotherapeutic agent for MMC (namely cisplatin [CDDP], as used with RT in squamous cell carcinoma of other sites, including head and neck, esophageal, and cervical cancers) could optimize the balance between disease-related outcomes and chemotherapy-related toxicities. These trials provided promising results for both CDDP as a substitute for MMC during CRT and CDDP-based induction chemotherapy prior to CRT.[19–21] These efforts prompted the remaining second-generation RCTs: RTOG 98-11, the UNICANCER ACCORD 03 trial, and the UKCCCR ACT II trial.[22–25] Despite the differences in study design and execution, all 3 of these RCTs sought to establish the role of CDDP as an alternative to MMC, as well as induction or maintenance chemotherapy in conjunction with CRT.

RTOG 98-11 randomized patients to RT + 5-FU/MMC versus induction 5-FU/CDDP followed by RT + 5-FU/CDDP. The study was terminated on interim analysis due to futility: the primary objective of improved 5-year DFS in the CDDP arm would not be met.[22] Furthermore, the initially reported results of RTOG 98-11 demonstrated significantly lower 5-year colostomy rates in the MMC arm (10% vs 19%).[22] Final reporting of the data for RTOG 98-11, shown in **Table 2**, demonstrated that the MMC arm had significantly better 5-year OS (78% vs 71%) and DFS (68% vs 58%), with trends toward better LRC (80% vs 74%) and CFS (72% vs 65%).[23] With regard to toxicity, the MMC arm experienced significantly higher grade 3 to 4 acute hematologic toxicity compared with the CDDP arm (62% vs 42%) but no difference in grade 3 to 4 acute nonhematologic (73% vs 72%) or grade 3 to 4 late toxicities (13% vs 11%).[23] Only 1 treatment-related fatality was reported, due to neutropenic sepsis, in the CDDP arm (N = 324).[23]

The ACCORD 03 trial evaluated a different approach, examining exclusively CDDP-based regimens and the roles of induction chemotherapy as well as higher-dose RT. This trial was predicated on phase II data supporting the use of induction (neoadjuvant) 5-FU/CDDP chemotherapy followed by CRT with 5-FU/CDDP.[24] The trial was also designed prior to the RTOG 98-11 results, which confirmed superiority of upfront CRT with MMC over induction CDDP-based chemotherapy followed by CDDP-based CRT. ACCORD 03 was designed as a 2 × 2 factorial RCT: all 4 arms received definitive treatment with 5-FU/CDDP concurrent with 45 Gy EBRT.[24] Arms A and B received induction chemotherapy (ICT) with 2 cycles of 5-FU/CDDP prior to

Table 2
Second-generation trial outcomes and toxicity profiles

Trial	Comparison	Disease-Related Outcomes				Acute Toxicities					Late Toxicities			
		Locoregional Control	Disease-free Survival	Overall Survival	Colostomy-free Survival	Hematologic	Skin	Gastrointestinal	Genitourinary	Other	Skin	Gastrointestinal	Genitourinary	Other
RTOG 87-04 (Flam et al,[18] 1996)	RT + 5-FU/MMC vs RT + 5-FU	84% vs 66%, 4 y. (LC)	73% vs 51%, 4 y	76% vs 67%, 4 y	71% vs 59%, 4 y	Grade 4-5: 18% vs 3%	Grade 4-5 nonhematologic toxicity: 7% vs 4%				Grade 4-5 late toxicity: 5% vs 1%			
RTOG 98-11 (Ajani et al,[22] 2008; Gunderson et al,[23] 2012)	RT + 5-FU/MMC vs Induction 5-FU/CDDP–CDDP > RT + 5-FU/CDDP	80% vs 74%, 5 y	68% vs 58%, 5 y	78% vs 71%, 5 y	72% vs 65%, 5 y	Grade 3-4: 62% vs 42%	Grade 3-4: 49% vs 41%	Grade 3-4: 37% vs 47%	Grade 3-4: 3% vs 3%	NR	Grade 3-4: 4% vs 2%	Grade 3-4: 3% vs 2%	NR	Total grade 3-4 Late toxicity: 13% vs 11%
ACCORD 03 (Peiffert et al,[24] 2012)	Induction 5-FU/CDDP– > RT + 5-FU/CDDP CRT vs RT + 5-FU/CDDP CRT	80% vs 81%, 5 y, (LC)	72% vs 65%, 5 y	72% vs 65%, 5 y	77% vs 75%, 5 y	Grade 3-4 (during CRT alone): 19% vs 12%	Grade 3-4 Mucositis (during CRT alone): 3% vs 3%	Grade 3-4 diarrhea (during CRT alone): 9% vs 11%	NR	NR	NR	Grade 3-4 diarrhea: 5%; grade 3-4 anal incontinence: 15%; grade 3-4 ulceration/fistula: 12% (all arms)	NR	Grade 3-4 bleeding: 25%; grade 3-4 anal pain: 12% (all arms)
ACT II (James et al,[25] 2013)	RT + 5-FU/MMC vs RT + 5-FU/CDDP	NR	69% vs 69%, 5 y	79% vs 77%, 5 y	68% vs 67%, 5 y	Grade 3-4 hematologic toxicity: 26% vs 16%; grade 3-4 leukopenia: 24% vs 12%; grade 3-4 febrile neutropenia: 3% vs 3%	Grade 3-4: 48% vs 47%	Grade 3-4: 16% vs 18%	Grade 3-4: 1% vs 2%	Grade 3-4 pain: 26% vs 29%	NR			

Abbreviation: NR, not reported.

definitive CRT (thus delaying CRT by 8 weeks); arms C and D received no ICT. After CRT, patients in arms A and C who responded to treatment received a standard RT boost of 15 Gy, whereas responders in arms B and D received high-dose RT boost of 20 Gy to 25 Gy; nonresponding patients in all arms proceeded to APR. The primary outcome measure of ACCORD 03 was CFS, and neither ICT nor higher-dose RT boost resulted in improved disease-related outcomes. ICT arms showed no improvement in CFS at 5 years (arms AB vs CD, 77% vs 75%) nor did the high-dose RT boost arms (arms BD vs AC, 78% vs 74%). Other disease-related outcomes, including DFS, OS, and LRC, were examined, and no significant differences were noted with either the addition of ICT or the higher-dose RT boost.[24] The investigators did not report toxicities by treatment arm, complicating interpretation of the ACCORD 03 data. The acute toxicity data reported, although not subjected to statistical analysis, compared ICT arms to CRT-alone arms (AB vs CD); these data suggested higher rates of grade 3 to 4 acute hematologic toxicity during CRT after ICT (19% vs 12%) (see **Table 2**). These figures also do not include the 15% of ICT patients who experienced grade 3 to 4 hematologic toxicity during ICT. It was further noted that ICT patients had 2-fold higher rates of chemotherapy-dose reduction related to toxicity during CRT (19% vs 9%). Late toxicities were not reported by treatment arm but rather by all patients pooled (see **Table 2**), with 1 to 3 treatment-related deaths occurring in each of the 4 treatment arms (N = 75–82 in each arm); no further details were provided regarding these events, making toxicity assessment in ACCORD 03 more difficult to interpret compared with concurrent RCTs.

Although ACCORD 03 focused on CDDP-based regimens, the last second-generation RCT, ACT II, evaluated MMC-based regimens as the standard approach. Given that the experimental arm of RTOG 98-11 combined both ICT and CDDP-based CRT, the trial left unanswered questions regarding the relative roles of ICT and CDDP-based CRT on outcomes and toxicity rates. To address these issues, ACT II was designed as a 2 × 2 factorial RCT: 1 randomization assigned patients to MMC-based or CDDP-based CRT, and a second assigned patients to receive adjuvant maintenance chemotherapy with 2 cycles of 5-FU/CDDP versus no maintenance therapy.[25] For the first randomization of MMC- versus CDDP-based CRT, the trial examined CR rates as well as acute toxicities with the 2 regimens (in the absence of subsequent maintenance therapy) as the primary endpoints. CR rates at 26 weeks from treatment initiation were similar for the MMC (91%) and CDDP (90%) CRT regimens. Furthermore, the overall acute toxicity profiles did not favor CDDP over MMC (total acute grade 3–4 toxicity, MMC vs CDDP, 71% vs 72%) (see **Table 2**). Acute hematologic toxicities were higher, however, in the MMC arm (grade 3–4, 26% vs 16%), due mostly to increased rates of neutropenia with MMC (grade 3–4, 24% vs 12%). Equal rates of febrile neutropenia were seen in the 2 arms (3% vs 3%). For the 2 non-maintenance arms (MMC and CDDP, each with N = 246), each arm had 1 treatment death within 4 weeks of treatment completion, and the MMC arm had 1 death 5 to 8 weeks after treatment completion due to non-neutropenic sepsis. Therefore, the higher hematologic toxicity rates with MMC did not translate into increased rates of neutropenic sepsis; given the challenges of CDDP administration (day-long infusion as opposed to 10-minute MMC delivery, requirements for concurrent intravenous hydration with CDDP, CDDP-related neuropathy risk), the investigators concluded that MMC should remain standard of care within the CRT regimen.[25]

The second ACT II treatment randomization (addition of 2 cycles of 5-FU/CDDP maintenance chemotherapy vs none) did not affect long-term disease-related outcomes. DFS at 3 years was no different with or without maintenance chemotherapy (74% vs 73%, respectively). Long-term disease related outcomes were also no different in the non-maintenance MMC and CDDP arms, respectively, including DFS, OS, and CFS (see **Table 2**). Late-term toxicity was not reported in the trial.[25] Collectively, ACT II demonstrated that maintenance therapy provided no outcomes benefits, and the standard of care for definitive management of anal cancer remains RT + 5-FU/MMC CRT.

Treatment Gap

One important issue raised by many of these trials is the significance of gaps, or delays in treatment. The ACT I, EORTC, and RTOG 87-04 trials all included a scheduled 4-week to 6-week treatment break after the initial 45 Gy, followed by RT boost, with boost dose determined by tumor response to initial treatment.[12,14,18] The ACCORD 03 trial similarly included a 3-week treatment gap between initial 45 Gy and boost delivery.[24] In contrast, RTOG 98-11 delivered a boost RT dose immediately following initial CRT for select patients, and ACT II consolidated all RT into a continuous 50.4 Gy regimen.[22,25] Multiple studies have sought to address what effects these variations in treatment course, including treatment breaks and boost doses, might have on outcomes. One analysis of the ACT I data suggested that the RT boost 6 weeks following the initial 45 Gy RT did not increase local control but rather increased late toxicity, in particular radionecrosis.[26] Another analysis, pooling the RTOG 87-04 and RTOG 98-11 trial data, demonstrated that total treatment duration was associated with higher rates of local failure as well as colostomy failure.[27] Two phase II trials further evaluated this issue. RTOG 92-08 attempted to deliver an escalated RT dose to 59.6 Gy using split course treatment (with a 2-week break during RT).[28] Comparing the patients of RTOG 92-08 to those of RTOG 87-04 (MMC arm), it was noted that the split course of treatment resulted in a lower incidence of grade 3 to 4 acute skin toxicity but markedly higher colostomy rates at 1 year (23% vs 6%) and 2 years (30% vs 7%). Long-term follow-up of RTOG 92-08 determined that split-course patients had low rates of late toxicity but lower DFS and CFS.[29] These conclusions were supported by ECOG 4292, another phase II dose-escalation trial, in which patients received 59.4 Gy either with or without a planned 2-week treatment break during RT. The cohort with the planned treatment break had markedly inferior 5-year OS (58% vs 84%) and progression-free survival (53% vs 85%) compared with the continuous cohort.[21] These data suggest improved disease-related outcomes with no planned treatment break. Along these lines, the absence of break or delay in the ACT II treatment scheme is regarded as one reason for the high CR and DFS rates relative to ACT I.[25] Despite the potential advantages of completing treatment without breaks, prior series have suggested that many patients require a break, and a small minority have to stop treatment entirely, both poor predictors of outcome.[27,29,30] Mitigating toxicities that lead to treatment breaks or cessation, therefore, is an important endpoint in optimizing outcomes. To that end, newer radiation techniques, in particular intensity-modulated RT (IMRT), have been implemented in the treatment of anal cancer.

PROSPECTS OF INTENSITY-MODULATED RADIOTHERAPY

Existing RCT data for anal cancer, from ACT I through ACT II, rely on older radiation techniques with homogenous radiation intensity in a given treatment field. These techniques, including 2-D (anteroposterior-posteroanterior [AP-PA]) RT or 3-D conformal RT (3D-CRT), deliver relatively high doses to tissues surrounding the treatment target. In contrast, IMRT allows for modulation of radiation intensity with a given field and often relies on a large number of fields for RT delivery (generally 9 or more fields for pelvic malignancies). In IMRT-based planning, strict radiation dose constraints to normal organs are established, doses are prescribed to different target volumes, and computer software inverse planning algorithms are used to design unconventional treatment fields that would not otherwise be possible with standard planning methods. IMRT involves partitioning of a given radiation field into multiple smaller fields, which can occur in the form of dynamic IMRT (in which collimating leaves, or blocks, move across an active radiation field using highly specific leaf sequences) or step-and-shoot IMRT (in which leaves sculpt the field shape while the beam is off). The end result of these approaches is that the intensity of the radiation beam for any one field varies. When these IMRT fields are summed, the cumulative effect is a radiation dose distribution that closely conforms the radiation dose around the tumor or target volumes while significantly reducing the dose to surrounding normal tissues. It was therefore postulated that IMRT might decrease toxicity by decreasing dose to surrounding normal tissues and consequently result in fewer treatment breaks as well as decreased overall treatment time.[31,32] Several single-arm retrospective (as well as a few prospective) series examined IMRT-based CRT in the definitive treatment of anal cancer, with lower rates of acute toxicities (primarily GI and skin) relative to the MMC arm of RTOG 98-11 as a 3D-CRT reference for comparison (**Table 3**).[33–45] Several series reported their institutional experiences comparing patients treated with 3D-CRT and IMRT, with similarly improved GI and skin toxicities (see **Table 3**).[46–50] As discussed elsewhere, these IMRT series report comparable disease-related outcomes compared with the MMC arm of RTOG 98-11.[10,51]

Despite this multitude of smaller experiences, only 1 phase II trial assessing the efficacy of IMRT has been conducted—RTOG 05-29. This study evaluated whether dose-painted IMRT (an approach whereby the primary/elective nodal target volumes as well as involved lymph nodes receive differing radiation doses synchronously using differing doses per fraction), with doses of 50.4 Gy to 54 Gy to the primary tumor, could reduce combined acute grade 2+ GU and GI toxicity compared with the MMC arm of RTOG 98-11 (which used 3D-CRT).[31] Although the primary endpoint was not met, the study did demonstrate significantly reduced grade 3+ dermatologic (23% vs 49%), grade 3+ GI (21% vs 36%), and grade 2+ hematologic (73% vs 85%) acute toxicity with IMRT versus 3D-CRT (see **Table 3**).[31] Additionally, fewer treatment breaks due to toxicity occurred with IMRT, consistent with other series demonstrating decreased treatment duration with the use of IMRT.[31,47–49] Collectively, with the reduction in GI and skin toxicities, and improved treatment tolerance, IMRT-based CRT has become a standard of care in the definitive treatment of anal cancer.[32]

Finally, the benefits of IMRT are predicated on reducing the dose delivered to organs at risk. Models supported by clinical data have determined that minimizing dose to organs at risk correlates with improved toxicity profiles. With regard to GI toxicity, for instance, one group reported that if a specific volume of small bowel receives less than 30 Gy, the rate of acute grade 3+ GI toxicity decreases 3-fold.[52] Similarly, other groups have provided dose constraints on the bony pelvis to minimize hematologic toxicity based on their dosimetric and clinical experience.[53–55] Atlases from both RTOG 05-29 and the Australasian Gastro-Intestinal Trials Group provide guidelines for IMRT contouring in the treatment of anal cancer.[31,56,57] The RTOG atlas in particular focuses on minimizing small bowel dose and consequently decreasing GI toxicity. Although these dosimetric constraints seem to translate into clinically significant improvements in toxicity, the caveat is that 81% of initially submitted IMRT plans for RTOG 05-29 patients required replanning, and 46% required multiple planning resubmissions.[31] These figures highlight the difficulty in quality assurance for IMRT-based studies and may account for the large variation in reported toxicity results with the use of IMRT across multiple institutions (see **Table 3**). They further serve to emphasize the increased complexity and cost associated with IMRT planning

Table 3
Acute toxicity profiles of intensity-modulated radiotherapy–based chemoradiation

Study	Notes	N	Acute Toxicities (Grade 3–4), %			
			Hematologic	Skin	Gastrointestinal	Genitorurinary
Prospective trials						
RTOG 98-11 (Ajani et al,[22] 2008; Gunderson et al,[23] 2012)	RT + 5-FU/MMC arm (RT with 3D-CRT for comparison)	325	62	49	37	3
RTOG 05-29 (Kachnic et al,[31] 2013)	IMRT + 5-FU/MMC	52	58	23	21	2
Single-arm IMRT series						
Milano et al,[33] 2005	(Retrospective)	17	53	0	0	0
Salama et al,[34] 2007	(Retrospective)	53	59	38	15	0
Pepek et al,[35] 2010	(Retrospective)	29	24	0	16	3
DeFoe et al,[36] 2012	(Retrospective)	78	13	29	28	NR
Kachnic et al,[37] 2012	(Retrospective)	43	51	10	7	7
Vieillot et al,[38] 2012	(Retrospective)	39	27	42	10	5
Han et al,[39] 2014	(Prospective)	58	41	46	9	0
Janssen et al,[40] 2014	(Retrospective)	25	19	24	0	0
Mitchell et al,[41] 2014	(Retrospective)	65	3	17	9	2
Belgioia et al,[42] 2015	(Retrospective)	41	5	5	7	0

Study	Design	N				
Franco et al,[43] 2015	(Prospective)	54	17	13	8	2
Yates et al,[44] 2015	(Retrospective)	42	19	33	14	NR
Call et al,[45] 2016	(Retrospective)	152	41	20	11	0
Comparison series						
Saarilahti et al,[46] 2008	(Retrospective, 3D-CRT vs IMRT)	39, 20 (3D-CRT, IMRT)	NR	82 vs 80	31 vs 0	35 vs 7
Bazan et al,[47] 2011	(Retrospective, 3D-CRT vs IMRT)	17, 29	29 vs 21	41 vs 21	29 vs 7	NR
Dewas et al,[48] 2012	(Retrospective, 3D-CRT vs IMRT)	27, 24	4 vs 4	35 vs 38	4 vs 4	NR
Chuong et al,[49] 2013	(Retrospective, 3D-CRT vs IMRT)	37, 52	38 vs 29 (leukopenia)	65 vs 12	30 vs 10	5 vs 0
Koerber et al,[50] 2014	(Retrospective, 3D-CRT vs IMRT)	37, 68	NR	95 vs 63 (grade 2–3)	68 vs 47 (grade 2–3)	NR

Abbreviations: N, number (of patients); NR, not reported.

compared with 3-D–CRT; one cost-effectiveness analysis, for instance, determined that the improved toxicity profile with IMRT was insufficient to outweigh the increased cost of IMRT.[58] Nevertheless, IMRT remains a standard approach in the definitive treatment of anal cancer owing to reduced toxicity rates.

MANAGEMENT OF TOXICITIES
Hematologic

As the progression of clinical trials illustrates, the acute hematologic toxicities associated with MMC have spurred efforts to find alternative agents; despite these efforts, MMC-based regimens remain the mainstay for definitive anal cancer treatment. Therefore, management of hematologic toxicities associated with MMC is critical. Particularly important are MMC dose-reduction protocols for patients with pre–MMC-dose leukopenia (<2400/μl) or thrombocytopenia (<85,000/μl); 2 of the 4 treatment-related deaths in the MMC arm of RTOG 87-04, all of which were due to neutropenia sepsis, were a result of nonadherence to dose reduction protocols.[18] Also, the MMC dosing paradigm differs by region, as previously discussed; comparisons of the 2-dose American MMC regimen and the 1-dose European MMC regimen have shown that the 2-dose regimen increases acute toxicities without improving outcomes, with increased hematologic and dermatologic toxicities as well as increased rates of hospitalizations due to febrile neutropenia.[59,60] Similarly, the use of single-dose MMC regimens may account for the improved acute grade 3 to 4 hematologic toxicity profile in ACT II versus RTOG 98-11 (see **Table 2**).[22,23,25] Further investigation is warranted into the efficacy and toxicity of these regimens, particularly with regard to the concentration of MMC dose as well as necessity for second dose delivery. Although these data support the use of single-dose MMC regimens, none explores the differential effects on outcome or toxicity with variable MMC doses, such as 10 mg/m^2 (per the RTOG studies), 12 mg/m^2 (per the ACT studies), or 15 mg/m^2 (per EORTC).[12,14,18,22,25,59,60] Lastly, guidelines regarding the prevention and management of chemotherapy-related myelosuppression and associated infection have been published extensively and are beyond the scope of this article.[61–63]

Gastrointestinal

Prevention and management of both acute and chronic GI side effects of pelvic RT have been a focus of recent research and reviews.[64–66] The most common acute GI toxicity, diarrhea, is typically managed with a combination of antidiarrheal agents (ie, loperamide and diphenoxylate/atropine), bulking agents, dietary modification, hydration and medication management (to minimize or substitute those medications that may promote diarrhea). A Cochrane review recently assess the role of dietary modification in minimizing acute diarrhea during pelvic RT and found that fat-restricted and fiber-supplemented diets may ameliorate diarrhea. The available literature, however, is prone to bias, and few RCTs have been conducted.[67] Several RCTs have assessed other interventions that seemed promising in smaller series but ultimately failed to improve acute GI toxicity in phase III trials. Two RCTs demonstrated that long-acting depot octreotide administration did not improve incidence or severity of acute diarrhea.[68,69] For both green tea tablets and statin medications, 1 RCT each has suggested benefit with regard to acute GI toxicity during pelvic RT.[70,71] In the absence of replicate data confirming these benefits, however, neither intervention has entered mainstream practice in the United States.

Common late GI toxicities of CRT for anal cancer include rectal bleeding and fecal incontinence.[64,66] Rectal bleeding, often a result of RT-induced telangiectasia development, is generally managed algorithmically, as previously reported, initially with endoscopic evaluation followed by bowel habit optimization and medical therapy.[64,66,72] Medical therapy options include sucralfate enemas and oral metronidazole with or without concurrent formalin therapy, all of which have been supported by small RCTs.[66,73–75] Although severe bleeding warrants urgent endoscopic management, chronic radiation proctitis has sometimes been treated with hyperbaric oxygen therapy.[64,66] This approach has recently been challenged, however, by publication of the HOT2 trial, a double-blind RCT evaluating hyperbaric oxygen for pelvic RT patients with late GI toxicities. In this study, hyperbaric oxygen therapy demonstrated no benefit in patients with chronic GI toxicities after pelvic RT, including rectal bleeding, and consequently the merits of hyperbaric oxygen in this setting have been questioned.[76] Fecal incontinence is typically managed with a combination of methods, including pelvic floor exercises, bulking agents, dietary modification, antidiarrheal medications, biofeedback techniques, surgical sphincter repair, and sacral nerve stimulation.[64,65] Short-term and long-term sacral nerve stimulation has shown some promise in decreasing episodes of fecal incontinence in small series, but these studies did not specifically examine patients with fecal incontinence after pelvic RT.[77,78] Finally, current efforts are exploring the role of radiation-induced gut microbiome changes, and the clinical benefits of altering intestinal flora to prevent or treat chronic RT-related GI toxicities.[79]

Dermatologic

Radiation dermatitis is common during pelvic RT for anal cancer and has been extensively discussed and reviewed previously.[80] Higher-grade (3–4) dermatitis can include severe moist desquamation or even skin ulceration and necrosis warranting grafting.[80] Prevention of severe dermatitis has sometimes involved use of topical moisturizers and antioxidants, such as aloe vera, whose efficacy in treating radiation dermatitis is supported by trial data.[81,82] Similarly, vigilant skin care and hygiene education during the treatment course can help minimize severity and avoid infection. Patient education in terms of practical lifestyle recommendations to prevent exacerbation of dermatitis is also important.[80]

Urinary

Urinary toxicities after CRT for anal cancer, although less frequent than GI toxicities, typically include urinary frequency (both diurnal and nocturnal), incontinence, urgency, and dysuria.[83] These effects are generally believed to be associated with RT-induced changes in pelvic floor muscle function.[84] Given the few data available for urinary toxicities specific to anal cancer treatment, urinary adverse effects of pelvic RT and their management are often extrapolated from prostate, rectal, and gynecologic malignancies.[85] Treatment of urinary toxicities often includes behavioral and physical therapies, such as pelvic floor muscle strengthening, bladder training, and biofeedback; medical therapies, such as bladder relaxants (ie, oxybutynin) can be used as well.[86] Additionally, promising data have been recently reported regarding injection of urethral bulking agents in women with RT-induced stress incontinence.[87]

Sexual

Although not often reported in large clinical trial data, sexual toxicities of definitive CRT for anal cancer have become increasingly apparent. Data from quality-of-life (QOL) series have demonstrated high rates of long-term sexual toxicity after CRT for anal cancer, often with more than 50% of patients reporting significant difficulty with their sex lives.[83,88–90] These adverse effects include decreased interest, dyspareunia, erectile dysfunction, and loss of feeling attractive, among others.[90] For women, vaginal stenosis causing dyspareunia is common after pelvic RT for anal cancer, causing grade 2 or higher stenosis in more than 60% of patients.[91] Efforts to both prevent and treat these symptoms center on combination usage of dilators, topical estrogen, and moisturizers/lubricants.[10,92] Another approach involves the use of sexual health counseling, validated by a recent RCT demonstrating improved psychological and sexual QOL metrics with such counseling sessions.[93] For men, phosphodiesterase inhibitors are typically used to improve sexual function. Referrals to therapists and counselors specializing in sexual health may be beneficial, as are considerations of patients' underlying psychological health and its role in sexual symptomatology.

Quality of Life

The QOL literature for anal cancer has grown in recent years.[90] In addition to specific toxicities discussed previously, patients' psychological, emotional, and financial health is increasingly studied, with 1 recent systemic review detailing current literature on the topic.[90] In the acute setting, data from ACCORD 03 demonstrated that patients' QOL metrics improved 2 months after treatment compared with pretreatment baseline.[94] It is long-term follow-up studies, however, that have highlighted survivorship issues facing anal cancer patients, from fatigue and social dysfunction to depression.[83,88,90,95] Further study into these complex sequelae of anal cancer diagnosis and treatment is warranted. Providers, meanwhile, should continue to assess and address these QOL issues in long-term follow-up.

FUTURE DIRECTIONS
Alternative Regimens and Techniques

Although this review has largely focused on phase III clinical trial data, smaller studies have explored alternative treatment options, with mixed results. With regard to systemic therapy, studies have attempted to determine the role of epidermal growth factor receptor (EGFR) inhibitors as well as other combinations of chemotherapeutics with RT. Biologic therapy with the addition of cetuximab (an EGFR-inhibiting monoclonal antibody) to CRT was assessed across multiple studies. Initial phase I data demonstrated unexpectedly high toxicity rates, including 1 study in which 26% of patients developed treatment-related thrombosis/embolism and another study which was closed prematurely due to serious adverse effects in 88% of treated patients.[96–98] Furthermore, long-term follow-up of one of these studies showed high rates of treatment failure, with approximately half of patients demonstrating disease relapse by 4-year follow-up.[99] Despite these setbacks, more promising results have been seen in preliminary results for the phase II ECOG E3205 and AMC-045 studies, which are examining the addition of cetuximab to CRT regimens in immunocompetent and HIV-positive patients, respectively.[100]

Other chemotherapy regimens have also been explored. One phase II EORTC trial assessed the use of CDDP/MMC-based CRT as opposed to 5-FU/MMC–based CRT and demonstrated prohibitive toxicity; approximately 30% of CDDP/MMC patients discontinued treatment due to toxicity, and less than half of these patients were fully compliant with treatment protocol, significantly worse than the 5-FU/MMC arm.[101] Phase II studies have also evaluated capecitabine-based regimens, serving as an oral fluoropyrimidine substitute for intravenous 5-FU. Early results indicate both low toxicity rates with acceptable outcomes using capecitabine/MMC-based and capecitabine/oxaliplatin-based CRT regimens, although these results have yet to be validated with larger studies.[102,103]

Building on the successes of IMRT, further advances in radiation technique and technology are also under investigation, with potential to reduce CRT-related toxicities while maintaining or improving disease-related outcomes. Volumetric-modulated arc therapy (VMAT) incorporates dynamic modulation of dose rate as radiation is delivered over an arc at approximately 180 positions around a patient, potentially resulting in a more efficient delivery of IMRT with decreased treatment times.[104] VMAT-based treatment of anal cancer has been successful in small series with improved toxicity profiles compared with 3D-CRT, but no clinical outcomes have compared traditional IMRT and VMAT.[105,106] Helical tomotherapy, in which small beams of radiation are delivered on a spiral around the patient, similarly represents an evolution of IMRT; recent series have begun to report outcomes with helical tomotherapy–based treatment of anal cancer, suggesting comparable toxicities and outcomes as with IMRT.[107,108] Proton beam therapy (PBT), in contrast to photon-based EBRT (including IMRT), has also been proposed to confer potential benefit in the treatment of anal cancer patients; PBT, due to its physical and dosimetric properties, allows for minimal dose delivery beyond the tumor volume in a given beam.[109,110] Dosimetric studies predict improve toxicities with PBT over IMRT, in particular hematologic and GI toxicities, as PBT reduces dose to the small bowel and marrow spaces, respectively.[109,110] Results of a prospective pilot study using PBT-based definitive CRT for anal cancer are anticipated within the near future.[111]

Future Clinical Trials

The next generation of clinical trials largely seeks to focus on personalizing treatment based on tumor properties. Along these lines, UK investigators are pursuing an umbrella phase II/III trial known as Personalising Anal Cancer Radiotherapy Dose (PLATO); within PLATO are the ACT III and ACT IV trials. Given that more advanced lesions (T3–4 tumors and node-positive) have higher rates of treatment failure, the PLATO trials stratify early-stage (T1 and T2 <4 cm N0) and late-stage (T3-4 [any N], T2N2–3) patients in the ACT III and ACT IV trials, respectively. ACT III returns back to the original data from the Nigro regimen, in which doses as low as 30 Gy were used effectively for early-stage disease.[7] This study will randomize patients to receive 50.4 Gy (ACT II dose) versus de-escalated 41.4 Gy, attempting to determine if the de-escalated arm results in improved toxicities while preserving LRC rates. In contrast, ACT IV emphasizes dose escalation for late-stage disease; this trial is predicated on results from the ACCORD 03 study, which demonstrated a nonsignificant trend toward improved CFS with high-dose RT boost.[24] Therefore, ACT IV will randomize patients to receive 53.2 Gy, 58.8 Gy, or 61.6 Gy, with a phase II/III design, assessing toxicity and complete response in the phase II, and LRC and acute/late toxicities in the phase III component.

Finally, given the role of oncogenic human papillomavirus (HPV) infection in anal intraepithelial neoplasia (AIN) and anal cancer, the role of vaccine therapy has also become a topic of investigation.[10] Vaccination against oncogenic strains of HPV have been shown to reduce the rates of AIN in one large RCT, and therefore use of the HPV vaccine to prevent anal cancer is an actively expanding field of study.[112] The Brown University Oncology Research Group evaluated the addition of 4 infusions of ADXS11-001, a bacteria-based vaccine targeting HPV-infected cells, with standard first-line IMRT + 5-FU/MMC.[113] Eligibility required tumors greater than 4 cm or node positive disease. Eleven patients have been entered since April 2013, including 6 with N2/3+ disease. Patients received the first vaccine infusion approximately 2 weeks before CRT, the second vaccine 10 to 28 days after completion of RT, and the third and fourth vaccines at subsequent monthly intervals. Three patients had grade 3 toxicities related to the vaccine, including chills/rigors (N = 2), back pain (N = 1), and hypokalemia (N = 1). All toxicities were within 24 hours of the immunotherapy infusion. There has been no enhancement of CRT toxicities (including myelosuppression) with ADXS11-001. All patients who have completed treatment on this pilot have had a clinical CR to vaccine therapy and CRT.[113]

SUMMARY

Over the past several decades, tremendous strides have been achieved in improving outcomes in the definitive management of anal cancer. However, the current standard of care, CRT with 5-FU/MMC, remains a toxic regimen despite providing high cure rates. Future directions are focusing on mitigating toxicities as well as optimizing survival and individualizing treatment approaches in anal cancer patients.

REFERENCES

1. Nelson RA, Levine AM, Bernstein L, et al. Changing patterns of anal canal carcinoma in the United States. J Clin Oncol 2013;31(12):1569–75.
2. Seigel RL, Miller KD, Jemal A. Cancer statistics, 2016. CA Cancer J Clin 2016; 66(1):7–30.
3. Boman BM, Moertel CG, O'Connell MJ, et al. Carcinoma of the anal canal. A clinical and pathologic study of 188 cases. Cancer 1984;54(1):114–25.
4. Frost DB, Richards PC, Montague ED, et al. Epidermoid cancer of the anorectum. Cancer 1984;53(6):1285–93.
5. Grabenbauer GG, Schneider IH, Gall FP, et al. Epidermoid carcinoma of the anal canal: treatment by combined radiation and chemotherapy. Radiother Oncol 1993;27(1):59–62.
6. Nigro ND, Vaitkevicius VK, Considine B Jr. Combined therapy for cancer of the anal cancer: a preliminary report. Dis Colon Rectum 1974;17(3):354–6.
7. Leichman L, Nigro N, Vaitkevicius S, et al. Cancer of the anal canal. Model for preoperative adjuvant combined modality therapy. Am J Med 1985;78(2):211–5.
8. Nigro ND, Vaitkevicius VK, Considine B Jr. Dynamic management of squamous cell cancer of the anal canal. Invest New Drugs 1989;7(1):83–9.
9. Benson AB 3rd, Arnoletti JP, Bekaii-Saab T, et al. Anal carcinoma, version 2.2012: featured updates to the NCCN guidelines. J Natl Compr Canc Netw 2012;10(4):449–54.
10. Shridhar R, Shibata D, Chan E, et al. Anal cancer: current standards in care and recent changes in practice. CA Cancer J Clin 2015;65(2):139–62.
11. Green JP, Schaupp WC, Cantril ST, et al. Anal carcinoma: current therapeutic concepts. Am J Surg 1980;140(1):151–5.
12. UKCCCR Anal Cancer Trial Working Party. Epidermoid anal cancer: results from the UKCCCR randomized trial of radiotherapy alone versus radiotherapy, 5-fluorouracil, and mitomycin. Lancet 1996;348(9034):1049–54.
13. Northover J, Glynne-Jones R, Sebag-Montefiore D, et al. Chemoradiation for the treatment of epidermoid anal cancer: 13-year follow-up of the first randomized UKCCCR Anal Cancer Trial (ACT I). Br J Cancer 2010;102(7):1123–8.
14. Bartelink H, Roelofsen F, Eschwege F, et al. Concomitant radiotherapy and chemotherapy is superior to radiotherapy alone in the treatment of locally advanced anal cancer: results of a phase III randomized trial of the European Organization for Research and Treatment of Cancer Radiotherapy and Gastrointestinal Cooperative Groups. J Clin Oncol 1997;15(5):2040–9.

15. Byfield JE, Barone RM, Sharp TR, et al. Conservative management without alkylating agents of squamous cell anal cancer using cyclical 5-FU alone and x-ray therapy. Cancer Treat Rep 1983;67(7–8):709–12.
16. Sischy B, Doggett RL, Krall JM, et al. Definitive irradiation and chemotherapy for radiosensitization in management of anal carcinoma: interim report on Radiation Therapy Oncology study no. 8314. J Natl Cancer Inst 1989;81(11):850–6.
17. Cummings BJ, Keane TJ, O'Sullivan B, et al. Epidermoid anal cancer: treatment by radiation alone or by radiation and 5-fluorouracil with and without mitomycin C. Int J Radiat Oncol Biol Phys 1991;21(5):1115–25.
18. Flam M, John M, Pajak TF, et al. Role of mitomycin in combination with fluorouracil and radiotherapy, and of salvage chemoradiation in the definitive nonsurgical treatment of epidermoid carcinoma of the anal canal: results of a phase III randomized intergroup study. J Clin Oncol 1996;14(9):2527–39.
19. Doci R, Zucali R, La Monica G, et al. Primary chemoradiation therapy with fluorouracil and cisplatin for cancer of the anus: results in 35 consecutive patients. J Clin Oncol 1996;14(12):3121–5.
20. Peiffert D, Giovannini M, Ducreux M, et al. High-dose radiation therapy and neoadjuvant plus concomitant chemotherapy with 5-fluorouracil and cisplatin in patients with locally advanced squamous-cell anal canal cancer: final results of a phase II study. Ann Oncol 2001;12(3):397–404.
21. Chakravarthy AB, Catalano PJ, Martenson JA, et al. Long-term follow-up of high-dose radiation with concurrent 5-fluorouracil and cisplatin in patients with anal cancer (ECOG E4292). Int J Radiat Oncol Biol Phys 2011;81(4):e607–13.
22. Ajani JA, Winter KA, Gunderson LL, et al. Fluorouracil, mitomycin, and radiotherapy vs fluorouracil, cisplatin, and radiotherapy for carcinoma of the anal canal: a randomized controlled trial. JAMA 2008;299(16):1914–21.
23. Gunderson LL, Winter KA, Ajani JA, et al. Long-term update of US GI intergroup RTOG 98-11 phase III trial for anal carcinoma: survival, relapse, and colostomy failure with concurrent chemoradiation involving fluorouracil/mitomycin versus fluorouracil/cisplatin. J Clin Oncol 2012;30(35):4344–51.
24. Peiffert D, Tournier-Rangeard L, Gérard JP, et al. Induction chemotherapy and dose intensification of the radiation boost in locally advanced anal canal carcinoma: final analysis of the randomized UNICANCER ACCORD 03 trial. J Clin Oncol 2012;30(16):1941–8.
25. James RD, Glynne-Jones R, Meadows HM, et al. Mitomycin or cisplatin chemoradiation with or without maintenance chemotherapy for treatment of squamous-cell carcinoma of the anus (ACT II): a randomised, phase 3, open-label, 2 × 2 factorial trial. Lancet Oncol 2013;14(6):516–24.
26. Glynne-Jones R, Sebag-Montefiore D, Adams R, et al. "Mind the gap"–the impact of variations in the duration of the treatment gap and overall treatment time in the first UK Anal Cancer Trial (ACT I). Int J Radiat Oncol Biol Phys 2011;81(5):1488–94.
27. Ben-Josef E, Moughan J, Ajani JA, et al. Impact of overall treatment time on survival and local control in patients with anal cancer: a pooled data analysis of Radiation Therapy Oncology Group trials 87-04 and 98-11. J Clin Oncol 2010;28(34):5061–6.
28. John M, Pajak T, Flam M, et al. Dose escalation in chemoradiation for anal cancer: preliminary results of RTOG 92-08. Cancer J Sci Am 1996;2(4):205–11.
29. Konski A, Garcia M Jr, John M, et al. Evaluation of planned treatment breaks during radiation therapy for anal cancer: update of RTOG 92-08. Int J Radiat Oncol Biol Phys 2008;72(1):114–8.

30. Roohipour R, Patil S, Goodman KA, et al. Squamous-cell carcinoma of the anal canal: predictors of treatment outcome. Dis Colon Rectum 2008;51(2):147–53.

31. Kachnic LA, Winter K, Myerson RJ, et al. RTOG 0529: a phase 2 evaluation of dose-painted intensity modulated radiation therapy in combination with 5-fluorouracil and mitomycin-C for the reduction of acute morbidity in carcinoma of the anal canal. Int J Radiat Oncol Biol Phys 2013;86(1):27–33.

32. Glynne-Jones R, Tan D, Hughes R, et al. Squamous-cell carcinoma of the anus: progress in radiotherapy treatment. Nat Rev Clin Oncol 2016;13(7):447–59.

33. Milano MT, Jani AB, Farrey KJ, et al. Intensity-modulated radiation therapy (IMRT) in the treatment of anal cancer: toxicity and clinical outcome. Int J Radiat Oncol Biol Phys 2005;63(2):354–61.

34. Salama JK, Mell LK, Schomas DA, et al. Concurrent chemotherapy and intensity-modulated radiation therapy for anal canal cancer patients: a multicenter experience. J Clin Oncol 2007;25(29):4581–6.

35. Pepek JM, Willett CG, Wu QJ, et al. Intensity-modulated radiation therapy for anal malignancies: a preliminary toxicity and disease outcomes analysis. Int J Radiat Oncol Biol Phys 2010;78(5):1413–9.

36. DeFoe SG, Deriwal S, Jones H, et al. Concurrent chemotherapy and intensity-modulated radiation therapy for anal carcinoma–clinical outcomes in a large National Cancer Institute-designated integrated cancer centre network. Clin Oncol (R Coll Radiol) 2012;24(6):424–31.

37. Kachnic LA, Tsai HK, Coen JJ, et al. Dose-painted intensity-modulated radiation therapy for anal cancer: a multi-institutional report of acute toxicity and response to therapy. Int J Radiat Oncol Biol Phys 2012;82(1):153–8.

38. Vieillot S, Fenoglietto P, Lemanksi C, et al. IMRT for locally advanced anal cancer: clinical experience of the Montpellier Cancer Center. Radiat Oncol 2012;7:45.

39. Han K, Cummings BJ, Lindsay P, et al. Prospective evaluation of acute toxicity and quality of life after IMRT and concurrent chemotherapy for anal canal and perianal cancer. Int J Radiat Oncol Biol Phys 2014;90(3):587–94.

40. Janssen S, Glanzmann C, Bauerfeind P, et al. Clinical experience of SIB-IMRT in anal cancer and selective literature review. Radiat Oncol 2014;9:199.

41. Mitchell MP, Abboud M, Eng C, et al. Intensity-modulated radiation therapy with concurrent chemotherapy for anal cancer: outcomes and toxicity. Am J Clin Oncol 2014;37(5):461–6.

42. Belgioia L, Vagge S, Agnese D, et al. Intensified intensity-modulated radiotherapy in anal cancer with prevalent HPV p16 positivity. World J Gastroenterol 2015;21(37):10688–96.

43. Franco P, Mistrangelo M, Arcadipane F, et al. Intensity-modulated radiation therapy with simultaneous integrated boost combined with concurrent chemotherapy for the treatment of anal cancer patients: 4-year results of a consecutive case series. Cancer Invest 2015;33(6):259–66.

44. Yates P, Carroll S, Kneebone A, et al. Implementing intensity-modulated radiotherapy with simultaneous integrated boost for anal cancer: 3 year outcomes at two Sydney Institutions. Clin Oncol (R Coll Radiol) 2015;27(12):700–7.

45. Call JA, Prendergast BM, Jensen LG, et al. Intensity-modulated radiation therapy for anal cancer: results from a Multi-Institutional Retrospective Cohort Study. Am J Clin Oncol 2016;39(1):8–12.

46. Saarilahti K, Arponen P, Vaalavirta L, et al. The effect of intensity-modulated radiotherapy and high dose rate brachytherapy on acute and late

radiotherapy-related adverse events following chemoradiotherapy of anal cancer. Radiother Oncol 2008;87(3):383–90.

47. Bazan JG, Hara W, Hsu A, et al. Intensity-modulated radiation therapy versus conventional radiation therapy for squamous cell carcinoma of the anal canal. Cancer 2011;117(15):3342–51.

48. Dewas CV, Maingon P, Dalban C, et al. Does gap-free intensity modulated chemoradiation therapy provide a greater clinical benefit than 3D conformal chemoradiation in patients with anal cancer? Radiat Oncol 2012;7:201.

49. Chuong MD, Freilich JM, Hoffe SE, et al. Intensity-modulated radiation therapy vs. 3D conformal radiation therapy for squamous cell carcinoma of the anal canal. Gastrointest Cancer Res 2013;6(2):39–45.

50. Koerber SA, Slynko A, Haefner MF, et al. Efficacy and toxicity of chemoradiation in patients with anal cancer–a retrospective analysis. Radiat Oncol 2014;9:113.

51. Zagar TM, Willett CG, Czito BG. Intensity-modulated radiation therapy for anal cancer: toxicity versus outcomes. Oncology (Williston Park) 2010;24(9):815–23.

52. Devisetty K, Mell LK, Salama JK, et al. A multi-institutional acute gastrointestinal toxicity analysis of anal cancer patients treated with concurrent intensity-modulated radiation therapy (IMRT) and chemotherapy. Radiother Oncol 2009;93(2):298–301.

53. Mell LK, Schomas DA, Salama JK, et al. Association between bone marrow dosimetric parameters and acute hematologic toxicity in anal cancer patients treated with concurrent chemotherapy and intensity-modulated radiotherapy. Int J Radiat Oncol Biol Phys 2008;70(5):1431–7.

54. Bazan JG, Luxton G, Mok EC, et al. Normal tissue complication probability modeling of acute hematologic toxicity in patients treated with intensity-modulated radiation therapy for squamous cell carcinoma of the anal canal. Int J Radiat Oncol Biol Phys 2012;84(3):700–6.

55. Julie DA, Oh JH, Apte AP, et al. Predictors of acute toxicities during definitive chemoradiation using intensity-modulated radiotherapy for anal squamous cell carcinoma. Acta Oncol 2016;55(2):208–16.

56. Myerson RJ, Garofalo MC, El Naqa I, et al. Elective clinical target volumes for conformal therapy in anorectal cancer: a radiation therapy oncology group consensus panel contouring atlas. Int J Radiat Oncol Biol Phys 2009;74(3):824–30.

57. Ng M, Leong T, Chander S, et al. Australasian Gastrointestinal Trials Group (AGITG) contouring atlas and planning guidelines for intensity-modulated radiotherapy in anal cancer. Int J Radiat Oncol Biol Phys 2012;83(5):145–62.

58. Hodges JC, Beg MS, Das P, et al. Cost-effectiveness analysis of intensity modulated radiation therapy versus 3-dimensional conformal radiation therapy for anal cancer. Int J Radiat Oncol Biol Phys 2014;89(4):773–83.

59. Yeung R, McConnell Y, Roxin G, et al. One compared with two cycles of mitomycin C in chemoradiotherapy for anal cancer: analysis of outcomes and toxicity. Curr Oncol 2014;21(3):e449–56.

60. White EC, Goldman K, Aleshin A, et al. Chemoradiotherapy for squamous cell carcinoma of the anal canal: comparison of one versus two cycles mitomycin-C. Radiother Oncol 2015;117(2):240–5.

61. Baden LR, Bensinger W, Angarone M, et al. Prevention and treatment of cancer-related infections. J Natl Compr Canc Netw 2012;10(11):1412–45.

62. Rodgers GM 3rd, Becker PS, Blinder M, et al. Cancer- and chemotherapy-induced anemia. J Natl Compr Canc Netw 2012;10(5):628–53.

63. Crawford J, Armitage J, Balducci L, et al. Myeloid growth factors. J Natl Compr Canc Netw 2013;11(10):1266–90.
64. Fuccio L, Guido A, Andreyev HJ. Management of intestinal complications in patients with pelvic radiation disease. Clin Gastroenterol Hepatol 2012;10(12): 1326–34.
65. Andreyev HJ, Muls AC, Norton C, et al. Guidance: the practical management of the gastrointestinal symptoms of pelvic radiation disease. Frontline Gastroenterol 2015;6(1):53–72.
66. Teo MT, Sebag-Montefiore D, Donnellan CF. Prevention and management of radiation-induced late gastrointestinal toxicity. Clin Oncol (R Coll Radiol) 2015; 27(11):656–67.
67. Henson CC, Burden S, Davidson SE, et al. Nutritional interventions for reducing gastrointestinal toxicity in adults undergoing radical pelvic radiotherapy. Cochrane Database Syst Rev 2013;(11):CD009896.
68. Martenson JA, Halyard MY, Sloan JA, et al. Phase III, double-blind study of depot octreotide versus placebo in the prevention of acute diarrhea in patients receiving pelvic radiation therapy: results of North Central Cancer Treatment Group N00CA. J Clin Oncol 2008;26(32):5248–53.
69. Zachariah B, Gwede CK, James J, et al. Octreotide acetate in prevention of chemoradiation-induced diarrhea in anorectal cancer: randomized RTOG trial 0315. J Natl Cancer Inst 2010;102(8):547–56.
70. Emami H, Nikoobin F, Roayaei M, et al. Double-blinded, randomized, placebo-controlled study to evaluate the effectiveness of green tea in preventing acute gastrointestinal complications due to radiotherapy. J Res Med Sci 2014;19(5): 445–50.
71. Wedlake LJ, Silia F, Benton B, et al. Evaluating the efficacy of statins and ACE-inhibitors in reducing gastrointestinal toxicity in patients receiving radiotherapy for pelvic malignancies. Eur J Cancer 2012;48(14):2117–24.
72. Andreyev HJ, Benton BE, Lalji A, et al. Algorithm-based management of patients with gastrointestinal symptoms in patients after pelvic radiation treatment (ORBIT): a randomised controlled trial. Lancet 2013;382(9910):2084–92.
73. Kochhar R, Patel F, Dhar A, et al. Radiation-induced proctosigmoiditis. Prospective, randomized, double-blind controlled trial of oral sulfasalazine plus rectal steroids versus rectal sucralfate. Dig Dis Sci 1991;36(1):103–7.
74. Cavcić J, Turcić J, Martinac P, et al. Metronidazole in the treatment of chronic radiation proctitis: clinical trial. Croat Med J 2000;41(3):314–8.
75. Sahakitrungruang C, Patiwongpaisarn A, Kanjanasilp P, et al. A randomized controlled trial comparing colonic irrigation and oral antibiotics administration versus 4% formalin application for treatment of hemorrhagic radiation proctitis. Dis Colon Rectum 2012;55(10):1053–8.
76. Glover M, Smerdon GR, Andreyev HJ, et al. Hyperbaric oxygen for patients with chronic bowel dysfunction after pelvic radiotherapy (HOT2): a randomised, double-blind, sham-controlled phase 3 trial. Lancet Oncol 2016;17(2):224–33.
77. Vaizey CJ, Kamm MA, Turner IC, et al. Effects of short term sacral nerve stimulation on anal and rectal function in patients with anal incontinence. Gut 1999; 44(3):407–12.
78. Malouf AJ, Vaizey CJ, Nicholls RJ, et al. Permanent sacral nerve stimulation for fecal incontinence. Ann Surg 2000;232(1):143–8.
79. Ferreira MR, Muls A, Dearnaley DP, et al. Microbiota and radiation-induced bowel toxicity: lessons from inflammatory bowel disease for the radiation oncologist. Lancet Oncol 2014;15(3):e139–47.

80. Fogh S, Yom SS. Symptom management during the radiation oncology treatment course: a practical guide for the oncology clinician. Semin Oncol 2014; 41(6):764–75.

81. Haddad P, Amouzgar-Hashemi F, Samsami S, et al. Aloe vera for prevention of radiation-induced dermatitis: a self-controlled clinical trial. Curr Oncol 2013; 20(4):e345–8.

82. Kodiyan J, Amber KT. Topical antioxidants in radiodermatitis: a clinical review. Int J Palliat Nurs 2015;21(9):446–52.

83. Bentzen AG, Balteskar L, Wanderås EH, et al. Impaired health-related quality of life after chemoradiotherapy for anal cancer: late effects in a national cohort of 128 survivors. Acta Oncol 2013;52(4):736–44.

84. Bernard S, Ouellet MP, Moffet H, et al. Effects of radiation therapy on the structure and function of the pelvic floor muscles of patients with cancer in the pelvic area: a systematic review. J Cancer Surviv 2016;10(2):351–62.

85. Liberman D, Mehus B, Elliott SP. Urinary adverse effects of pelvic radiotherapy. Transl Androl Urol 2014;3(2):186–95.

86. Michaelson MD, Cotter SE, Gargollo PC, et al. Management of complications of prostate cancer treatment. CA Cancer J Clin 2008;58(4):196–213.

87. Krhut J, Martan A, Jurakova M, et al. Treatment of stress urinary incontinence using polyacrylamide hydrogel in women after radiotherapy: 1-year follow-up. Int Urogynecol J 2016;27(2):301–5.

88. Das P, Cantor SB, Parker CL, et al. Long-term quality of life after radiotherapy for the treatment of anal cancer. Cancer 2010;116(4):882–9.

89. Knowles G, Haigh R, McLean C, et al. Late effects and quality of life after chemo-radiation for the treatment of anal cancer. Eur J Oncol Nurs 2015; 19(5):479–85.

90. Sodergren SC, Vassiliou V, Dennis K, et al. Systematic review of the quality of life issues associated with anal cancer and its treatment with radiochemotherapy. Support Care Cancer 2015;23(12):3613–23.

91. Mirabeau-Beale K, Hong TS, Niemierko A, et al. Clinical and treatment factors associated with vaginal stenosis after definitive chemoradiation for anal canal cancer. Pract Radiat Oncol 2015;5(3):e113–8.

92. Cullen K, Fergus K, Dasgupta T, et al. Toward clinical care guidelines for supporting rehabilitative vaginal dilator use with women recovering from cervical cancer. Support Care Cancer 2013;21(7):1911–7.

93. DuHamel K, Schuler T, Nelson C, et al. The sexual health of female rectal and anal cancer survivors: results of a pilot randomized psycho-educational intervention trial. J Cancer Surviv 2016;10(3):553–63.

94. Tournier-Rangeard L, Mercier M, Peiffert D, et al. Radiochemotherapy of locally advanced anal canal carcinoma: prospective assessment of early impact on the quality of life (randomized trial ACCORD 03). Radiother Oncol 2008;87(3): 391–7.

95. Welzel G, Hägele V, Wenz F, et al. Quality of life outcomes in patients with anal cancer after combined radiochemotherapy. Strahlenther Onkol 2011;187(3): 175–82.

96. Olivatto LO, Vieira FM, Pereira BV, et al. Phase 1 study of cetuximab in combination with 5-fluorouracil, cisplatin, and radiotherapy in patients with locally advanced anal canal carcinoma. Cancer 2013;119(16):2973–80.

97. Deutsch E, Lemanski C, Pignon JP, et al. Unexpected toxicity of cetuximab combined with conventional chemoradiotherapy in patients with locally advanced

anal cancer: results of the UNICANCER ACCORD 16 phase II trial. Ann Oncol 2013;24(11):2834–8.

98. Leon O, Guren MG, Radu C, et al. Phase I study of cetuximab in combination with 5-fluorouracil, mitomycin C and radiotherapy in patients with locally advanced anal cancer. Eur J Cancer 2015;51(18):2740–6.

99. Levy A, Azria D, Pignon JP, et al. Low response rate after cetuximab combined with conventional chemoradiotherapy in patients with locally advanced anal cancer: long-term results of the UNICANCER ACCORD 16 phase II trial. Radiother Oncol 2015;114(3):415–6.

100. Garg M, Lee JY, Kachnic LA, et al. Phase II trials of cetuximab (CX) plus cisplatin (CDDP), 5-fluorouracil (5-FU) and radiation (RT) in immunocompetent (ECOG 3205) and HIV-positive (AMC045) patients with squamous cell carcinoma of the anal canal (SCAC): Safety and preliminary efficacy results. J Clin Oncol 2012;30(S15) [abstract: 4030].

101. Matzinger O, Roelofsen F, Mineur L, et al. Mitomycin C with continuous fluorouracil or with cisplatin in combination with radiotherapy for locally advanced anal cancer (European Organisation for Research and Treatment of Cancer phase II study 22011-40014). Eur J Cancer 2009;45(16):2782–91.

102. Glynne-Jones R, Meadows H, Wan S, et al. EXTRA–a multicenter phase II study of chemoradiation using a 5 day per week oral regimen of capecitabine and intravenous mitomycin C in anal cancer. Int J Radiat Oncol Biol Phys 2008; 72(1):119–26.

103. Eng C, Chang G, Das P, et al. Phase II study of capecitabine and oxaliplatin with concurrent radiation therapy (XELOX-XRT) for squamous cell carcinoma of the anal canal. J Clin Oncol 2009;27(S15) [abstract: 4116].

104. Mok H, Briere TM, Martel MK, et al. Comparative analysis of volumetric modulated arc therapy versus intensity modulated radiation therapy for radiotherapy of anal carcinoma. Pract Radiat Oncol 2011;1(3):163–72.

105. Weber HE, Dröge L, Hennies S, et al. Volumetric intensity-modulated arc therapy vs. 3-dimensional conformal radiotherapy for primary chemoradiotherapy of anal carcinoma: effects on treatment-related side effects and survival. Strahlenther Onkol 2015;191(11):827–34.

106. Franco P, Arcadipane F, Ragona R, et al. Volumetric modulated arc therapy (VMAT) in the combined modality treatment of anal cancer patients. Br J Radiol 2016;89(1060):20150832.

107. Joseph K, Nijjar Y, Warkentin H, et al. Prospective phase II study of tomotherapy based chemoradiation treatment for locally advanced anal cancer. Radiother Oncol 2015;117(2):234–9.

108. Vendrely V, Henrigues de Figueiredo B, Rio E, et al. French multicentre clinical evaluation of helical TomoTherapy for anal cancer in a cohort of 64 consecutive patients. Radiat Oncol 2015;10:170.

109. Anand A, Bues M, Rule WG, et al. Scanning proton beam therapy reduces normal tissue exposure in pelvic radiotherapy for anal cancer. Radiother Oncol 2015;117(3):505–8.

110. Ojerholm E, Kirk ML, Thompson RF, et al. Pencil-beam scanning proton therapy for anal cancer: a dosimetric comparison with intensity-modulated radiotherapy. Acta Oncol 2015;54(8):1209–17.

111. Wo J, Ben-Josef E. A pilot feasibility study of definitive concurrent chemoradiation with pencil beam scanning proton beam in combination with 5-fluorouracil and mitomycin-C for carcinoma of the anal canal. Available at: https://clinicaltrials.gov/ct2/show/NCT01858025. Accessed February 21, 2016.

112. Palefsky JM, Guiliano AR, Goldstone S, et al. HPV vaccine against anal HPV infection and anal intraepithelial neoplasia. N Engl J Med 2011;365(17): 1576–85.
113. Perez K, Safran H, Leonard K, et al. ADXS11-001 immunotherapy with chemo-radiation for anal cancer. Int Anal Neoplasia Soc Presented. Atlanta (GA), March 13, 2015.

Locally Recurrent Disease Related to Anal Canal Cancers

Tarik Sammour, MBChB, FRACS, PhD, Miguel A. Rodriguez-Bigas, MD, John M. Skibber, MD*

KEYWORDS

- Anal cancer • Anal squamous cell carcinoma • Anal canal • Local recurrence
- Exenteration

KEY POINTS

- Less than 20% of patients suffer locoregional failure after chemoradiation therapy for anal cancer.
- Complete restaging with MRI pelvis and computed tomography–positron emission tomography followed by multidisciplinary tumor board discussion is required in all patients considered for surgery.
- The ability to achieve R0 resection with acceptable morbidity determines the potential for salvage surgery, which may involve extensive resection of perineal soft tissue and/or pelvic organs with subsequent reconstruction.
- In patients planned for curative resection, an R0 resection is ultimately achieved in the majority of patients (86%), with 5 year overall and disease-free survival of 60%.
- Careful patient selection, and shared decision making in a specialized multidisciplinary setting is paramount for achieving acceptable patient-centered outcomes.

INTRODUCTION

Chemoradiation therapy (CRT) is the standard of care in the primary treatment of anal squamous cell carcinoma (SCC), with salvage surgery reserved for the less than 20% of patients who suffer locoregional failure with persistent disease (within 6 months) or recurrent disease (after 6 months).[1,2] There are several factors that can predict failure, the most obvious being a higher T stage or N stage,[2] with a reported one-third of

Disclosure Statement: The authors have nothing to disclose.
Division of Surgery, Department of Surgical Oncology, The University of Texas MD Anderson Cancer Center, 1400 Pressler Street, P.O. Box 301402, Houston, TX 77230-1402, USA
* Corresponding author. Department of Surgical Oncology, The University of Texas MD Anderson Cancer Center, Room Number: FCT17.6032, P.O. Box 301402, Unit 1484, Houston, TX 77030-1402.
E-mail address: jskibber@mdanderson.org

patients with T4 or N3 disease developing a local recurrence. Of patients who develop locoregional failure, 75% involve the anus or rectum; 20% recur elsewhere in the pelvis outside the radiotherapy field, and less than 5% recur in the inguinal nodal basins.[2]

A vital component for the management of these patients is early detection of recurrences. Because biopsy of the post-CRT scar is no longer routinely recommended because of poor yield, and there is no reliable tumor marker to measure, detection of recurrences is heavily reliant on detailed clinical follow-up.[3] This entails a detailed physical examination with a digital rectal examination, anoscopy, and inguinal palpation for nodal involvement, as well as protocolized cross-sectional imaging for surveillance of more advanced disease.

If a local recurrence is detected, then complete restaging is required followed by multidisciplinary discussion and consideration for salvage surgery.

SURGICAL TECHNIQUE
Preoperative Planning

History
A full account of the patient's medical, surgical, and social history is obtained. Several points are of specific importance in the setting of locally recurrent anal cancer:

- Does the patient have pain, weight loss; leg swelling; neurologic, obstructive, and/or urinary symptoms; or gynecologic symptoms in females? Importantly, symptoms present at the time of diagnosis may have implications for resectability and prognosis.[4]
- When and where were the primary CRT treatments undertaken? Details of doses, radiation fields, duration, and patient tolerance are required to enable planning of future CRT regimens.
- Review of histology.
- What is the patient's human immunodeficiency virus (HIV) status, human papilloma virus (HPV) status, and details of immunization?
- What postoperative surveillance has the patient undergone so far? Details of serial examination, anoscopy, nodal assessment, and cross-sectional imaging are useful to indicate rate of progression.
- Review of systems to enable determination of medical fitness for further treatment.
- Social history including functional status, cognitive ability, quality of life, social support, and patient preferences are required to facilitate shared decision-making discussions.

Examination
Digital rectal examination to document the precise tumor location and extent, and to establish involvement of adjacent structures, as well as palpation of nodal basins is required. In female patients, a per-vaginal examination can also help to determine vaginal involvement. Rectal and vaginal examination may have to be performed in the operating room under general anesthetic if discomfort does not permit adequate assessment in the outpatient setting, and this may also allow confirmatory biopsy if this has not been done. Finally, assessment of the abdominal wall, looking specifically for incisional hernia and the state of the rectus abdominis muscle on both sides is important if there is likely to be a need for soft tissue reconstruction. For the same reason, the state of the perineum after radiotherapy should also be assessed.

Imaging

The purpose of cross-sectional imaging is to establish 2 important facts regarding the anatomy of the recurrence that will determine whether curative treatment is an option:

Whether there is distant metastatic disease
Local resectability (predicted R0 resection)

Multiphase contrast-enhanced computed tomography (CT) of the chest, abdomen, and pelvis is commonly used for the detection of metastatic tumor deposits. In some institutions, including the authors' institution, fluorodeoxyglucose [18F] positron emission tomography with CT (PET/CT) is utilized routinely as part of the initial assessment of recurrent disease, as there is some evidence that it alters management in a significant subset of patients (**Fig. 1**).[5] High-resolution MRI with or without diffusion weighted imaging (DWI) is the current standard of care for evaluation of pelvic resectability.[6] Good-quality T2-weighted images are essential (see **Fig. 1**), preferably accompanied by standardized reporting with specific comment on the involvement of any pelvic viscera and nodal disease (**Fig. 2**).

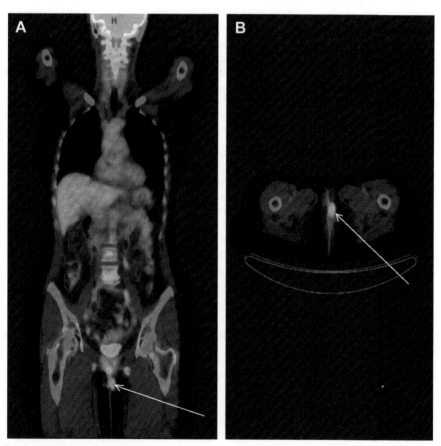

Fig. 1. PET/CT scan demonstrating area of active anal squamous cell carcinoma recurrence in the left perineal region (*arrow*).

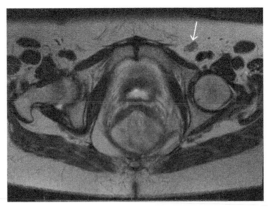

Fig. 2. MRI scan demonstrating involved left inguinal lymph node in the setting of recurrent anal squamous cell carcinoma.

Multidisciplinary considerations

After the previously described assessment and investigations are performed, the patient's case is reviewed at a multidisciplinary tumor board meeting, and the options for management are discussed. In the absence of distant metastatic deposits, treatment with curative intent mandates surgical resection of all known disease. Most commonly this will mean an abdominoperineal resection, but treatment can range from repeat wide local excision (rarely) to complete pelvic exenteration with multivisceral resection, sacrectomy, and reconstruction.

Patients with locally recurrent anal cancer with pelvic disease should only be offered exenterative surgery if all of the following criteria are fulfilled:

1. Complete R0 resection is technically possible based on imaging.
   a. Absolute technical contraindications to resection are: unresectable extrapelvic disease, para-aortic node involvement, bilateral sciatic nerve involvement, circumferential bone involvement, lumbar spine involvement (above L5/S1).
   b. Relative contraindications are: tumor extension through the sciatic notch, encasement of external iliac vessels, and high sacral involvement (sacrectomy above S2/S3 junction is controversial but can be performed in selected centers).
2. The patient is medically fit to undergo the procedure.
3. The patient is cognitively able to engage in a shared decision making discussion, and give reasonable informed consent.

If the patient is not a candidate for exenterative surgery, then a palliative surgical option would be proximal fecal diversion if soiling or feculent vaginal discharge is an issue. A loop sigmoid colostomy via a minimally invasive surgical approach is ideal if this is technically achievable.

Informed consent

After multidisciplinary tumor board recommendations have been finalized, a face-to-face meeting between the primary colorectal surgeon and the patient accompanied by a support person (such as a close family member) is scheduled to facilitate formal discussion and informed consent. There may me multiple options offered to the patient, and each of these needs to be discussed fully, outlining the benefits and risks. The consent discussion should also include details of planned stomas and the possibility of the surgeon finding unexpected metastatic disease intraoperatively that is unresectable and would lead to the procedure being aborted. A shared decision-making process on the part of the attending surgeon and the patient is required and should be clearly documented.

It is usual for the patient to also discuss management with a medical oncologist, a radiation oncologist, and any other surgical services that are expected to be involved during the operation. Involvement of a cancer nurse specialist or care coordinator, an ostomy nurse, and relevant allied health staff such as cultural support workers and interpreters is prudent.

Medical optimization

Given the magnitude of the surgery to be undertaken, the management of all relevant medical comorbidities should be optimized, with the help of perioperative care physicians and the involvement of anesthetists, preferably with experience in this type of surgery. In patients who require it based on screening assessments, preoperative nutritional support and prehabilitation programs should be undertaken.[7] There is a high risk of intraoperative hemorrhage, and any anticoagulants the patient is on preoperatively should be managed accordingly. Wound healing or lack thereof is a common postoperative concern, and preoperative smoking cessation is actively encouraged, especially if flap closure is planned.

Coordination of multidisciplinary team

Depending on the anatomy of the surgery to performed, a multidisciplinary team of surgeons may be required. Anticipated involvement based on preoperative assessment should result in the patient being seen and consented by the relevant service ahead of time in the outpatient setting. Pelvic and perineal defects may require flap closure by a plastic surgeon. Less commonly, such as in the setting of pelvic disease require exenteration, involvement of urologists, vascular surgeons, and orthopedic surgeons may be required.

The patient should be marked by an experienced stoma nurse to facilitate assessment of stoma location in standing, supine, and sitting positions, and when the patient is in his or her usual clothes. Given the lengthy nature of this type of surgery, it is important that delays are minimized by effective coordination.

Preparation and Patient Positioning

The patient is usually placed in modified Lloyd-Davies position, with provision for undertaking part of the procedure via a perineal or posterior approach if necessary. Calf compression devices and precautions against pressure areas are routinely used. A folded towel or roll may be placed under the sacrum to improve access to the perineum. The whole perineum including the anal region and vagina in females is prepped. Prepping and draping should take into account not only the needs of the primary surgeon, but also the optimal exposure and preparation for the other members of the multidisciplinary surgical team. For example, if an inguinal lymphadenectomy is to be performed, then the inguinal region needs to be exposed appropriately.

Surgical Approach

Exploration and/or wide local excision

The first step is digital rectal examination and vaginal examination in women to re-establish the anatomy of the disease. If the recurrence is localized without significant anal sphincter involvement, then a perineal-only approach such as a repeat wide local excision with or without flap closure may be all that is required. However, if the disease is more advanced, then an abdominoperineal resection is usually required.

Abdominal phase

An exploratory laparotomy is performed first. All 4 quadrants of the abdomen, including the liver, the diaphragm, and the small and large bowel and their mesentery are visually inspected and palpated. A finding of unexpected metastatic disease that is unresectable should be confirmed with intraoperative frozen section, and the procedure should be abandoned save for palliative defunctioning stoma if deemed beneficial by the operating surgeon. In the absence of unresectable metastatic disease, the next step is a complete adhesiolysis, followed by mobilization of the sigmoid colon and left colon. The left ureter is identified and preserved. The splenic flexure is not routinely mobilized, but this may be required for added length to facilitate end colostomy formation. The inferior mesenteric artery is then identified and isolated. This is secured and divided where feasible for length and the ends ligated with a heavy braided absorbable suture. The inferior mesenteric vein is identified and isolated. This is secured and divided where feasible for length, with the ends ligated with a heavy braided absorbable suture. A high tie of the inferior mesenteric vessels is not usually required from an oncological point of view, but may be needed to achieve adequate length on the stoma, particularly in overweight patients.

Pelvic phase

Rectal dissection is undertaken in the total mesorectal excision (TME) plane. The point of division of the inferior mesenteric artery leads the surgeon into the plane posteriorly, and dissection is continued distally as far as possible. Lateral dissection and anterior dissection are then completed, and circumferential TME is completed down to the pelvic floor.

Exenteration

In patients with more advanced disease, extended resection may be required, most commonly including posterior colpectomy for women[8] or a partial prostatectomy for men.[9] In the 20% of patients with pelvic recurrence, pelvic exenteration is required. Identification of any normal uninvolved planes and dissecting within these are usually the best place to start. Dissection then continues from easier and softer tissues toward more difficult and rigid areas, with wider margins taken as necessary. Identification of the ureters and a decision regarding whether one or both can be preserved can often be the defining step in this operation. Ureteric catheters are a useful aid to assist in palpation and identification of the ureters, which, if free, can be slung with a vascular loop and preserved. Options for ureteric reconstruction include uretero-ureterostomy with or without psoas hitch, ureteric reimplantation, or Boari flap repair. If the situation is not directly reconstructable, then the urologist may proceed with a radical cystectomy with out without prostatectomy and subsequent ileal or colonic conduit reconstruction after the specimen is removed.

In cases with extensive lateral pelvic sidewall involvement, iliac vessel identification and dissection are required. If the common, external, or internal iliac arteries or veins are invaded by tumor, then en bloc resection and reconstruction by a vascular surgeon may be considered to achieve R0 resection, although this is done highly selectively.[10] First, the internal iliac artery and its branches are ligated distal to the superior gluteal artery to minimize buttock claudication and preserve supply to any potential gluteal flaps. Lymph node dissection is performed including nodal tissue overlying the aortoiliac bifurcation down to the origin of the internal iliac. Proximal control and distal control of the internal iliac vein are achieved, and smaller branches are divided prior to division of the main trunk. The lateral and middle sacral vein branches are also ligated and divided, and dissection is continued along the pelvic sidewall bilaterally down to the pelvic floor, with the dissection completed from below if required. Extended lateral pelvic sidewall excision, including resection of the sciatic nerve, has also been described.[11]

En bloc sacrectomy can also be performed if necessary with orthopedic surgeon involvement. Resections above S3 require conversion to the prone position, whereas below S3 a combined abdominal/perineal approach can be used.[12] All gluteus muscular attachments to the posterior aspect of the coccyx and sacrum are dissected free up to a point above the planned site of sacral transection. The sacrococcygeal ligaments are divided off the sacrum, and the anterior sacrum is scored with diathermy at the level of planned transection. Division is possible with the patients still in the supine position using 2 osteotomes, one placed posterior to the sacrum to protect the skin and the other anteriorly for transection. For sacrectomy above the level of S3, temporary or permanent closure of the abdomen is required prior to turning the patient prone, and the sacrectomy is completed from below.

If possible, an omental pedicle flap based on the right gastroepiploic artery is fashioned and used to fill the dead space in the pelvis.[9] A rectus abdominis muscle-only flap can also be used to achieve this. At least 1 intra-abdominal drain is often used and placed in the pelvis as well.

Perineal phase

This component of the resection is highly variable, and dependent on the extent of local perineal disease. The general over-riding principle is wide local excision of the perineal component of the recurrent tumor with clear margins, which often requires complete excision of the anal sphincter complex. In women, vaginal recurrence is common, and therefore, posterior vaginectomy should be considered.[8] At times anterior extension to include en bloc resection of the urogenital organs is warranted.

Intraoperative radiotherapy

Any margins that are not obviously macroscopically clear are confirmed with intraoperative frozen section. Intraoperative radiotherapy (IORT) is administered selectively with consultation with the radiation oncologist if any resection margins are microscopically positive (R1) based on intraoperative frozen pathology assessment, or if the margins were negative but 2 mm or less.[13,14] At the authors' center, IORT is administered using high-dose rate iridium-192 brachytherapy using a Harrison–Anderson–Mick applicator, with a dose of 10 to 15 Gy at 1 cm from the radiation source.[15]

Ilioinguinal lymphadenectomy

A small subset of patients recur in the ilioinguinal nodal basins, and can undergo lymph node dissection with good outcomes.[16] A folded towel is placed behind the pelvis on the affected side, with the ipsilateral hip slightly flexed and laterally rotated to maximize exposure. If a laparotomy was already performed, then iliac lymph node dissection can be performed through this incision. Inguinal lymphadenectomy requires a separate incision over the femoral triangle. If a laparotomy has not been performed, then an S-shaped incision is made from the anterior superior iliac spine to the apex of the femoral triangle with the oblique part of the incision in the groin crease. This allows access to both the iliac and inguinal compartments. The inguinal ligament is identified and divided, and this incision is extended vertically into the external oblique aponeurosis. The spermatic cord is retracted medially, and the internal oblique/transversus muscles are divided. The inferior epigastric vessels are ligated and divided. The peritoneum, bladder, and rectum are retracted medially. The superior limit of dissection is the common iliac artery overlying the sacroiliac joint. Lymph node dissection begins laterally on the pelvic sidewall and progresses medially, with all lymphatic tissue surrounding the external iliac vessels, obturator canal, and internal iliac vessels retrieved.

Dissection then continues inferiorly into the inguinal compartment progressing from superficial tissues to deep. The great saphenous vein is identified and ligated flush onto the femoral vein at the saphenofemoral junction. Dissection of all lymphatic tissue from the lateral border of sartorius muscle to the medial border of gracilis muscle is performed. Centrally, a block of nodal tissue is dissected off the femoral artery and vein, which are skeletonized to the floor of the femoral triangle. Femoral canal nodes are included in this part of the specimen. Inferiorly, the dissection continues down to the apex of the femoral triangle, at which point the more proximal aspect of the great saphenous vein is ligated and divided.

Soft tissue reconstruction

The size of the defect depends on the extent of the resection (determines anteropos-terior and lateral dimensions), and the patient's body habitus (determines depth). The complexity of the reconstruction can be compounded by the presence of stomas, pre-vious incisions, and hernias, as well as vascular supply to tissue flaps or lack thereof. Close consultation with experienced plastic surgical services is therefore required at all stages.

Flap closure of perineal defects reduces wound complications compared with at-tempts at primary closure, particularly after radiation treatment.[17,18] It is possible to use absorbable or biological mesh to reconstruct the pelvic floor, but this technique may still require additional soft tissue coverage, as primary skin closure is not always possible without tension.[19] Selection of which flap to use is based on the size of the defect, the availability of tissue, the characteristics of the patient, and the local exper-tise available. The most common technique utilized for perineal reconstruction is the vertical rectus abdominis myocutaneous flap (VRAM) based on the inferior epigastric artery, which is a robust flap that usually affords significant tissue bulk.[20] Harvesting of this flap leaves a defect in the anterior abdominal wall that usually requires repair with synthetic mesh or component separation techniques.[21] Other options include: gracilis muscle flaps,[22] inferior gluteal artery myocutaneous flaps (IGAM),[23] gluteal fold flaps,[24] anterolateral thigh flaps,[25] and full-thickness local advancement flaps.[26] In fe-male patients, vaginal reconstruction can be attempted using modifications of the pre-viously mentioned flaps, or including local rotation flaps such a modified Singapore flap.[27] A Sartorius muscle flap may be used to cover the femoral triangle compartment if this was dissected.

Immediate Postoperative Care

All patients are managed in a high-dependency unit setting immediately after surgery and transitioned to standard ward care as able. Principles of enhanced recovery after surgery are applied as closely as possible, while taking into account the magnitude of surgery undertaken, and the unique considerations that go along with this.[28] Wound complications are common in the setting of flap closure, particularly given the previ-ously irradiated tissue in this setting. This issue needs to be anticipated and actively managed.

REHABILITATION AND RECOVERY

Depending on the extent of the surgery, the rehabilitation process may be prolonged. The most common scenario involves an abdomino-perineal resection with flap closure. This necessitates stoma management and wound care teaching. Involvement of specialist stoma and wound care nurses, and an experienced physiotherapy service

Table 1
Summary of the selected recent data on long-term survival after planned curative surgery for recurrent anal cancer

Author, Year	n	R0	5 y OS	5 y DFS
Hannes et al,[31] 2016	14	86%	64%	86%
Severino et al,[3] 2016	25	64%	nr	nr
Lefevre et al,[9] 2012	55	nr	60%	48%
Mariani et al,[1] 2008	42	98%	61%	nr
Mullen et al,[32] 2007	20	nr	60%	nr
Ghouti et al,[33] 2005	21	nr	72%	48%
Akbari et al,[16] 2004	33	nr	51%	58%
Nilsson et al,[30] 2002	14	86%	82%	79%
Total/median	224	86%	61%	58%

Abbreviations: 5 y DFS, 5-year disease-free survival for all patients (R0, R1, R2); 5 y OS, 5-year overall survival for all patients (R0, R1, R2); n, number of planned curative resections; nr, not reported.

is prudent. Many patients have significant pain that is directly attributable to the neoplastic process or to the surgery itself. This symptom alone can become a major determinant of quality of life, and should be aggressively managed.[4]

CLINICAL RESULTS IN THE LITERATURE

The literature on management of anal cancer recurrence is limited to retrospective reviews with relatively small numbers (**Table 1**).[29] The median 5-year overall and disease-free survival in patients undergoing planned curative resection is approximately 60%, and an R0 resection is achievable in the majority of patients (86%). Prognostic factors for survival and recurrence are T status and the presence of an involved margin.[9] Other factors include the presence of metastatic lymph nodes (LNs), and neurolymphovascular invasion (NLVI).[3] Patients with local recurrence seem to have a better prognosis than those with persistent disease after CRT, presumed to be due to the more indolent biological behavior of the disease.[16,30]

SUMMARY

Surgery for anal cancer is usually reserved for patients with persistent disease or local recurrence after definitive CRT, which accounts for less than 20% of patients undergoing treatment. An important component of management is early detection of recurrences, and this is reliant on intensive clinical follow-up, particularly in high-risk cases. Patients with local recurrence should be re-evaluated fully for evidence of metastatic disease using PET-CT, and the local anatomy should be delineated with MRI. Eligible patients should undergo tailored surgery with the aim of achieving an R0 resection, which may require extensive resection of perineal soft tissue and/or pelvic organs with subsequent reconstruction. Given the heterogeneity of presentation and the morbidity of the surgery, management is best undertaken within a specialized multidisciplinary setting. In patients planned for curative resection, an R0 resection is ultimately achieved in the majority of patients (86%), with 5-year overall and disease-free survival of 60%. Careful patient selection and shared decision making are paramount for achieving acceptable patient-centered outcomes.

REFERENCES

1. Mariani P, Ghanneme A, De la Rochefordiere A, et al. Abdominoperineal resection for anal cancer. Dis Colon Rectum 2008;51(10):1495–501.
2. Das P, Bhatia S, Eng C, et al. Predictors and patterns of recurrence after definitive chemoradiation for anal cancer. Int J Radiat Oncol Biol Phys 2007;68(3):794–800.
3. Severino NP, Chadi SA, Rosen L, et al. Survival following salvage abdominoperineal resection for persistent and recurrent squamous cell carcinoma of the anus: do these disease categories affect survival? Colorectal Dis 2016. [Epub ahead of print].
4. You YN, Habiba H, Chang GJ, et al. Prognostic value of quality of life and pain in patients with locally recurrent rectal cancer. Ann Surg Oncol 2011;18(4):989–96.
5. Jones M, Hruby G, Solomon M, et al. The role of FDG-PET in the initial staging and response assessment of anal cancer: a systematic review and meta-analysis. Ann Surg Oncol 2015;22(11):3574–81.
6. Gourtsoyianni S, Goh V. MRI of anal cancer: assessing response to definitive chemoradiotherapy. Abdom Imaging 2014;39(1):2–17.
7. Gupta R, Gan TJ. Preoperative nutrition and prehabilitation. Anesthesiology Clin 2016;34(1):143–53.
8. Skibber J, Rodriguez-Bigas MA, Gordon PH. Surgical considerations in anal cancer. Surg Oncol Clin N Am 2004;13(2):321–38.
9. Lefevre JH, Corte H, Tiret E, et al. Abdominoperineal resection for squamous cell anal carcinoma: survival and risk factors for recurrence. Ann Surg Oncol 2012; 19(13):4186–92.
10. Solomon MJ, Brown KG, Koh CE, et al. Lateral pelvic compartment excision during pelvic exenteration. Br J Surg 2015;102(13):1710–7.
11. Shaikh I, Aston W, Hellawell G, et al. Extended lateral pelvic sidewall excision (EL-SiE): an approach to optimize complete resection rates in locally advanced or recurrent anorectal cancer involving the pelvic sidewall. Tech Coloproctol 2015; 19(2):119–20.
12. Solomon MJ, Tan KK, Bromilow RG, et al. Sacrectomy via the abdominal approach during pelvic exenteration. Dis Colon Rectum 2014;57(2):272–7.
13. Wright JL, Gollub MJ, Weiser MR, et al. Surgery and high-dose-rate intraoperative radiation therapy for recurrent squamous-cell carcinoma of the anal canal. Dis Colon Rectum 2011;54(9):1090–7.
14. Hallemeier CL, You YN, Larson DW, et al. Multimodality therapy including salvage surgical resection and intraoperative radiotherapy for patients with squamous-cell carcinoma of the anus with residual or recurrent disease after primary chemoradiotherapy. Dis Colon Rectum 2014;57(4):442–8.
15. You YN, Skibber JM, Hu CY, et al. Impact of multimodal therapy in locally recurrent rectal cancer. Br J Surg 2016. [Epub ahead of print].
16. Akbari RP, Paty PB, Guillem JG, et al. Oncologic outcomes of salvage surgery for epidermoid carcinoma of the anus initially managed with combined modality therapy. Dis Colon Rectum 2004;47(7):1136–44.
17. Khoo AK, Skibber JM, Nabawi AS, et al. Indications for immediate tissue transfer for soft tissue reconstruction in visceral pelvic surgery. Surgery 2001;130(3): 463–9.
18. Davidge KM, Raghuram K, Hofer SO, et al. Impact of flap reconstruction on perineal wound complications following ablative surgery for advanced and recurrent rectal cancers. Ann Surg Oncol 2014;21(6):2068–73.

19. Jensen KK, Rashid L, Pilsgaard B, et al. Pelvic floor reconstruction with a biological mesh after extralevator abdominoperineal excision leads to few perineal hernias and acceptable wound complication rates with minor movement limitations: single-centre experience including clinical examination and interview. Colorectal Dis 2014;16(3):192–7.
20. Touny A, Othman H, Maamoon S, et al. Perineal reconstruction using pedicled vertical rectus abdominis myocutaneous flap (VRAM). J Surg Oncol 2014; 110(6):752–7.
21. Campbell CA, Butler CE. Use of adjuvant techniques improves surgical outcomes of complex vertical rectus abdominis myocutaneous flap reconstructions of pelvic cancer defects. Plast Reconstr Surg 2011;128(2):447–58.
22. Chong TW, Balch GC, Kehoe SM, et al. Reconstruction of Large Perineal and Pelvic Wounds Using Gracilis Muscle Flaps. Ann Surg Oncol 2015;22(11):3738–44.
23. Boccola MA, Rozen WM, Ek EW, et al. Inferior gluteal artery myocutaneous island transposition flap reconstruction of irradiated perineal defects. J Plast Reconstr Aesthet Surg 2010;63(7):1169–75.
24. Pantelides NM, Davies RJ, Fearnhead NS, et al. The gluteal fold flap: a versatile option for perineal reconstruction following anorectal cancer resection. J Plast Reconstr Aesthet Surg 2013;66(6):812–20.
25. Wong S, Garvey P, Skibber J, et al. Reconstruction of pelvic exenteration defects with anterolateral thigh-vastus lateralis muscle flaps. Plast Reconstr Surg 2009; 124(4):1177–85.
26. Tashiro J, Yamaguchi S, Ishii T, et al. Salvage total pelvic exenteration with bilateral v-y advancement flap reconstruction for locally recurrent rectal cancer. Case Rep Gastroenterol 2013;7(1):175–81.
27. Woods JE, Alter G, Meland B, et al. Experience with vaginal reconstruction utilizing the modified Singapore flap. Plast Reconstr Surg 1992;90(2):270–4.
28. Stone AB, Grant MC, Pio Roda C, et al. Implementation Costs of an Enhanced Recovery After Surgery Program in the United States: A Financial Model and Sensitivity Analysis Based on Experiences at a Quaternary Academic Medical Center. J Am Coll Surg 2016;222(3):219–25.
29. Leon O, Guren M, Hagberg O, et al. Anal carcinoma - survival and recurrence in a large cohort of patients treated according to Nordic guidelines. Radiother Oncol 2014;113(3):352–8.
30. Nilsson PJ, Svensson C, Goldman S, et al. Salvage abdominoperineal resection in anal epidermoid cancer. Br J Surg 2002;89(11):1425–9.
31. Hannes S, Reinisch A, Bechstein WO, et al. Salvage abdominoperineal excisions in recurrent anal cancer-impact of different reconstruction techniques on outcome, morbidity, and complication rates. Int J Colorectal Dis 2016;31(3): 653–9.
32. Mullen JT, Rodriguez-Bigas MA, Chang GJ, et al. Results of surgical salvage after failed chemoradiation therapy for epidermoid carcinoma of the anal canal. Ann Surg Oncol 2007;14(2):478–83.
33. Ghouti L, Houvenaeghel G, Moutardier V, et al. Salvage abdominoperineal resection after failure of conservative treatment in anal epidermoid cancer. Dis Colon Rectum 2005;48(1):16–22.

Surveillance of Anal Canal Cancers

Richard Adams, BSc, BM BS, MRCP, FRCR, MD

KEYWORDS

- Anal cancer • Follow-up • Surveillance • Radical treatment • Salvage
- Squamous cell cancer

KEY POINTS

- Patients with radically treated anal canal squamous cell cancer (SCC) require surveillance/follow-up to allow salvage surgery to take place with the aim of cure in patients with persistent or locally recurrent disease.
- Clinical evaluation is critical with documentation of abnormalities that persist; continuity of care may assist in this process.
- Acute toxicities can be severe and must be managed after treatment to prevent escalation.
- Late toxicities relating to prior tumor-related damage and radiotherapy-related long-term side effects should be managed actively with specialist referral as appropriate.

INTRODUCTION

Patients with anal SCC treated with radical intent using CRT generally have an excellent prognosis. The US Radiotherapy Oncology Group 9811 trial (completed in 2005) indicates a 5-year overall survival rate of 75%.[1] There are more than 8000 new cases of anal cancer diagnosed per year in the United States.[2] With a majority of these patients treated with radical intent and an expected follow-up time of 5 years with low attrition, this may equate to greater than 25,000 patients who remain on active surveillance at any one point and an even larger number alive and in remission beyond 5 years.

Surveillance is a routine part of the management of most patients treated radically for cancer but it remains important to understand the rationale and basis for this practice in each cancer subtype.

Broadly, surveillance should aim to deliver:

- Timely interventions that have an impact on an individual's chances of cure or life prolongation.

Disclosure Statement: The author has nothing to disclose.
Division of Cancer and Genetics, Velindre Cancer Centre, Cardiff University, Whitchurch, Cardiff CF14 2TL, UK
E-mail address: richard.adams@wales.nhs.uk

Surg Oncol Clin N Am 26 (2017) 127–132
http://dx.doi.org/10.1016/j.soc.2016.07.007

- Improved quality of life, through:
  - Effective management of toxicities to prevent escalation
  - Psychological reassurance

When specifically looking at anal cancer, these factors can be mapped into the areas indicated in **Box 1**.

Although acknowledging that surveillance can offer significant psychological reassurance, this can result in marked anxieties around the time of the follow-up appointment or scan with a significant impact on an individual's quality of life.

This article explores these phenomena, the evidence, where available, and a rational approach where not.

CLINICAL GUIDELINES

International and national clinical guidelines are regularly updated and offer clinicians a benchmark by which to formulate their practice. Surveillance has infrequently been explored, however, in a rigorous fashion and thus levels of evidence are based on retrospective review and expert opinion.

The European Society for Medical Oncology (ESMO) and National Comprehensive Cancer Network (NCCN) guidelines[3,4] are probably the most frequently referred to internationally for many cancers, including anal cancer. Both sets of guidelines are similarly aligned but it is acknowledged that there is limited evidence on which to base their recommendations.

There are notable differences between these guidelines, as indicated in **Table 1**.

TIMING OF SURVEILLANCE

Early evaluation is based on 3 key factors:

1. The ability to formally clinically assess the anal canal by digital rectal examination (DRE) at a time when acute toxicities are regressing. Most patients are reasonably comfortably evaluable by the 8-week mark after CRT, although earlier evaluation to ensure symptom control ahead of this time should be tailored to the individual.
2. The knowledge that after completion of CRT, SCC of the anal canal may take many months to reach a nadir, including clinical complete response.
3. Rarer relapses after 3 years surveillance.

The often slow regression of tumor after completion of CRT is based on evidence from trials, such as anal cancer trial (ACT) II, in which randomized patients had trial-based documentation of clinical complete response at 11 weeks and 26 weeks post-completion of CRT. Data from this trial indicate that 29% of patients who did not demonstrate a complete remission at 11 weeks had achieved a complete response by 26 weeks, with durable response.[5]

Box 1
Key areas relevant to surveillance after radical treatment of anal squamous cell carcinoma

- Detection and monitoring of persistent disease after completion of radical CRT
- Detection of locoregional recurrent disease after radical CRT
- Management of acute/late toxicities
- Psychological reassurance

Table 1
A comparison of international guidelines for surveillance after radical treatment of anal
cancer: National Comprehensive Cancer Network and European Society for Medical Oncology

	European Society for Medical Oncology Guidelines	National Comprehensive Cancer Network Guidelines
Early clinical surveillance: timing	Initial evaluation at 8 wk after completion of CRT. Then 3–6 monthly for those in complete remission for a period of 2 y.	Initial evaluation at 8–12 wk after completion of CRT. Then 3–6 monthly for those in complete remission.
Late surveillance: timing	6–12 Monthly until 5 y	3–6 Monthly until 5 y
Clinical assessment at each visit to include	• DRE and palpation of the inguinal lymph nodes • Anoscopy or proctoscopy (optional, sometimes poorly tolerated and too painful after CRT)	• DRE and palpation of the inguinal lymph nodes • Anoscopy
Imaging recommendations	Possibly: MRI on a 6-mo basis for 3 y for locoregional assessment CT scans for distant recurrence are not currently recommended	Chest/abdomen/pelvic imaging annually for 3 y (if T3-T4 or inguinal node positive)
Persisting disease	Avoid biopsy for persisting disease at 8–12 wk evaluation up to 6 mo post-CRT	Re-evaluate 4 weekly until remission up to 6 mo post-CRT

Retrospective review of the phase III trials of radical CRT in anal cancer indicate that a majority of relapses and thus the most efficient time for more frequent surveillance are within the first 3 years of completion of CRT. The ACT II trial with long-term follow-up demonstrated less than 1% of relapses occurring beyond 3 years (**Fig. 1**).[5] Other trials suggest this may be closer to 5%; thus, there seems to be some rationale to continue surveillance out to 5 years.

CLINICAL EVALUATION

Clinical evaluation revolves around locoregional assessment.

Although many patients with earlier-stage disease have a return to a normal-feeling anal canal mucosa, those with more advanced initial disease, especially T3-T4 disease, often have residual changes and scarring even in the absence of residual tumor. Those patients with residual changes require consistent follow-up with good documentation of the changes identified. Any new thickening, growth, or ulceration should be evaluated. Examination under anesthetic (EUA) and potential targeted biopsy should be considered by a surgeon with experience in this disease.

DRE and potential use of anoscopy offer an ability beyond that offered by imaging to assess local disease persistence or recurrence. These can also give critical information relating to functional difficulties causing significant effects on quality of life, which may then be amenable to targeted intervention. Regional relapse can, at least in part, be assessed with inguinal nodal examination. As discussed previously, EUA should be reserved for those with persistent abnormalities 5 to 6 months after CRT, stenosis, pain, or scarring that prevents effective examination or new changes arising during surveillance.

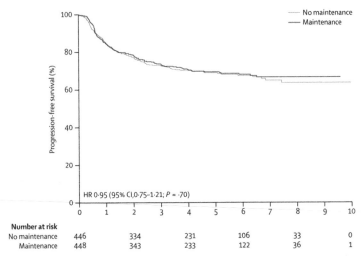

Fig. 1. Kaplan-Meier curves showing progression free survival in the ACT II trial of radical CRT for anal cancer. HR, hazard ratio. (*From* James RD, Glynne-Jones R, Meadows HM, et al. Mitomycin or cisplatin chemoradiation with or without maintenance chemotherapy for treatment of squamous-cell carcinoma of the anus [ACT II]: a randomised, phase 3, open-label, 2 × 2 factorial trial. Lancet Oncol 2013;14(6):519; with permission.)

It is widely acknowledged that locally persistent or recurrent disease can be salvaged surgically with curative intent with abdominoperineal excision with flap reconstruction and permanent stoma formation. Recent data seem to suggest that those patients with later relapse locally may have a better prognosis than those persisting or recurring early.[6]

Within the Severino and colleagues[6] data set, 36 patients underwent salvage abdomino-perineal resection for persistent or recurrent invasive cancer: 80.5% (29) had tumor identified on DRE, 13.9% (5) required EUA due to pain or stenosis, and in 5% (2), tumor was identified by imaging with no evident tumor on DRE. Three patients had disease identified in the inguinal nodes. All patients had biopsy-confirmed recurrence prior to salvage. In this data set, early disease was associated with later recurrence and those with persistent disease, which was more frequently of later stage, had the worst prognosis. Surgical salvage can result in durable survival. This series demonstrated a 3-year overall survival of 46%, which reaches approximately 90% in the late recurring disease group. A similar analysis has been performed on the patients from the ACT II trials in which 103 patients underwent surgical salvage; these data reveal similar results (Glynne Jones, personal communication, abstract submitted American Society of Clinical Oncology, 2016).

IMAGING RECOMMENDATIONS

There is little evidence in terms of optimized surveillance radiologic imaging. This is manifest in the differing recommendations from ESMO and NCCN (see **Table 1**).

To the authors' knowledge, no good data exist that early identification of distant metastatic disease is of any benefit to the patient. Individual case reports identify positive outcomes from isolated metastectomies or stereotactic radiotherapy for oligometastatic disease but are rare and inevitably these reports suffer from positive reporting bias. There are no data to indicate that early intervention in the palliative setting with chemotherapy improves outcome, although with the evolving interest in immunotherapies, such as the immune checkpoint inhibitors and tumor vaccines, it is rational that a low burden of disease may respond more effectively and durably.

A recent international survey involving 149 clinicians who specialize in anal cancer indicates that 87% routinely arrange surveillance imagining in the first 2 years; 18% of these were with CT/PET (all within the United States) and 21% with MRI, predominantly in Europe.[7] The variation seen in response to this questionnaire in itself underlines the uncertainty in this area but also indicates the allegiance to more regional guidelines.

MRI of the pelvis in line with pretreatment staging seems to be evolving as a relevant investigation to assess for locoregional relapse that may offer an earlier ability to salvage, although its strength in identifying anal canal recurrence remains limited compared with clinical evaluation.

The ESMO and NCCN guidelines for surveillance after radical CRT for cervix cancer are more relaxed in terms of their recommendations. In terms of recommending imaging only, if symptomatically indicated, ESMO cervix cancer surveillance guidelines state, "No definitive agreement exists on the best post-treatment surveillance...CT or PET/CT scan should be performed as clinically indicated."[8] NCCN cervix cancer surveillance guidelines state, "Imaging chest radiography, CT, PET-CT, MRI as indicated based upon symptoms or examination findings suspicious for recurrence but not recommended for routine surveillance, a single PET-CT performed at 3–6 months after CRT for locally advanced cervical cancer can be used to assess early or asymptomatic persistence or recurrence."[9]

SUMMARY

The surveillance of patients who have been treated radically with CRT for anal canal SCC is based on limited evidence. The guidelines that exist, however, are broadly based on sound principles. The major focus is on optimizing the opportunities for surgical salvage of persistent or locoregionally recurrent disease, with the aim of cure.

There is increasing interest in using the surveillance period to optimize quality of life; addressing significant late toxicities (addressed in allied chapter).

To date there is little to recommend a hunt for distant metastatic disease during this surveillance period and limited evidence to indicate a group of patients who are fit and do not warrant continued review over 5 years.

REFERENCES

1. Ajani JA, Winter KA, Gunderson LL, et al. Fluorouracil, mitomycin, and radiotherapy vs fluorouracil, cisplatin, and radiotherapy for carcinoma of the anal canal: a randomized controlled trial. JAMA 2008;299(16):1914–21.
2. Available at: http://www.cancer.org/acs/groups/content/@research/documents/document/acspc-047079.pdf. Accessed April 1, 2016.
3. Glynne-Jones R, Nilsson PJ, Aschele C, et al. Anal cancer: ESMO-ESSO-ESTRO Clinical Practice Guidelines for diagnosis, treatment and follow-up. Ann Oncol 2014;25(Suppl 3):iii10–20.
4. Available at: http://www.nccn.org/professionals/physician_gls/PDF/anal.pdf. Accessed April 1, 2016.
5. James RD, Glynne-Jones R, Meadows HM, et al. Mitomycin or cisplatin chemoradiation with or without maintenance chemotherapy for treatment of squamous-cell carcinoma of the anus (ACT II): a randomised, phase 3, open-label, 2 × 2 factorial trial. Lancet Oncol 2013;14(6):516–24.

6. Severino N, Chadi S, Rosen L, et al. Survival following salvage abdominoperineal resection for persistent and recurrent squamous cell carcinoma of the anus; do these disease categories affect survival Survival following salvage abdominoperineal resection for persistent and recurrent squamous cell carcinoma of the anus: do these disease categories affect survival? Colorectal Dis 2016. http://dx.doi.org/10.1111/codi.1328.
7. Eng C, Adams R, Kachnic L, et al, on behalf of the International Rare Cancer Initiative (IRCI) Working Group. Post-treatment surveillance in locally advanced squamous cell carcinoma (SCCA) of the anal canal: a global subspecialist survey. J Clin Oncol 2016;34(Suppl 4S):573 [abstract].
8. Colombo N, Carinelli S, Colombo A, et al, on behalf of the ESMO Guidelines Working Group Cervical cancer. ESMO Clinical Practice Guidelines for diagnosis, treatment and follow-up. Ann Oncol 2012;23(Supplement 7):vii27–32.
9. Available at: http://www.nccn.org/professionals/physician_gls/PDF/cervical.pdf. Accessed August 13, 2016.

Metastatic Anal Cancer and Novel Agents

Van Morris, MD, Cathy Eng, MD*

KEYWORDS

- Anal cancer • Squamous cell • Chemotherapy • Immunotherapy • HPV • PD-1

KEY POINTS

- Squamous cell carcinoma of the anal canal (SCCA) is a rare, understudied disease that can be cured by concurrent chemoradiation in the nonmetastatic setting.
- No consensus standard-of-care approach to the treatment of metastatic SCCA exists to date; cytotoxic doublet chemotherapeutic doublets have traditionally been utilized for metastatic disease.
- Early results from trials incorporating immune checkpoint blockade agents for the treatment of metastatic SCCA hold great promise for improving survival outcomes for patients with this disease.

INTRODUCTION

Anal cancer represents a rare disease that accounts for approximately 2% of all gastrointestinal (GI) malignancies.[1] Although most patients will present with locoregional disease, a fraction of patients will develop distant metastases.[2–4] This article focuses on the management of metastatic disease of anal cancers of squamous cell histology and not of other underlying histologies like adenocarcinoma or anal melanoma. Previous experiences with systemic chemotherapies and local therapies for oligometastases will be discussed, as will the role of emerging immunotherapy agents as a novel approach to the treatment of distant metastases.

EPIDEMIOLOGY

Over 90% of anal cancers are of squamous cell histology. In 2016, it is estimated that over 8000 new cases of squamous cell carcinoma of the anal canal (SCCA) will be diagnosed in the United States, with over 1000 deaths from this disease.[1] The annual incidence of SCCA continues to rise, both in the United States and globally, and it is

The authors have nothing to disclose.
Department of Gastrointestinal Medical Oncology, The University of Texas – MD Anderson Cancer Center, 1515 Holcombe Boulevard, Unit 426, Houston, TX 77030, USA
* Corresponding author.
E-mail address: ceng@mdanderson.org

surgonc.theclinics.com

expected that this trend will continue for decades to come.[5] Risk factors for the development of anal cancer include a prior history of gynecologic malignancy, tobacco use, a history of multiple sexual partners, and impaired immunity, whether from use of immunosuppressive agents, underlying autoimmune disease, or from coexisting human immunodeficiency virus/acquired immunodeficiency syndrome (HIV/AIDS).[6–10]

However, by far the most prevalent factor responsible for the development of SCCA is coinfection with human papilloma virus (HPV).[8,11,12] This virus also plays an important role in other malignancies such as squamous cell carcinoma of the head and neck, cervical cancer, vaginal/vulvar cancer, and penile cancer.[13–20] Incorporation of viral DNA into the host cell genome results in expression of the viral oncoproteins E6 and E7, which disrupt p53 and Rb, respectively, to promote oncogenesis.[21–23] In a series of patients with metastatic SCCA treated at the authors' institution, the presence of HPV, assessed by the detection of HPV by DNA in situ hybridization and/or p16 by immunohistochemistry, occurred in over 95% of tested tumors.[24] Other groups have also reported that most anal cancers are associated with HPV infection,[25,26] and it appears as though the presence of HPV serves as a positive prognostic biomarker from these reports, a trend that is similar to outcomes in other HPV-associated malignancies.

HPV-16 is the most common subtype of HPV associated with the development of SCCA.[27] In recent years, preventative quadrivalent and nonavalent vaccines against the most common subtypes of HPV have been introduced to children and adolescents with no prior HPV exposure. Initial reports with this primary prevention approach in adolescent girls have suggested success rates in lowering the incidence of precancerous cervical lesions.[28,29] Applied to SCCA, 1 prospective study demonstrated that, in a population of men who have-sex with men, use of preventative vaccines against HPV led to lower rates of anal dysplasia.[30] These data have not fully matured to demonstrate lower rates of anal cancer with such vaccines, although updated results are greatly anticipated. The authors suspect that in the decades to come, a generalized trend toward decreased prevalence/incidence of SCCA will occur as the result of these HPV vaccines.

MANAGEMENT OF LOCOREGIONAL SQUAMOUS CELL CARCINOMA OF THE ANAL CANAL

Most patients with newly diagnosed SCCA will present with locoregional disease that has not spread to distant organs. For these patients, the standard of care approach has not changed for decades. Here, patients receive concurrent chemoradiation with either 5–FU/mitomycin C or with 5–FU/cisplatin.[31–35]

Although concurrent chemoradiation is successful in curing SCCA in the majority of patients, approximately 10% to 30% of this population will develop a locoregional failure with recurrent disease at the site of the primary tumor.[2,36] Risk factors for recurrence include a primary tumor greater than 5 cm in longest dimension, the presence of regional lymph nodes at diagnosis, and male gender.[3] For such patients who recur after chemoradiation, the standard of care is abdominoperineal resection (APR),[36] which has a success rate with respect to 5-year survival of approximately 40% to 65% following surgery, despite the presence of a tumor that was not eradicated upfront by chemoradiation.[37–39]

MANAGEMENT OF METASTATIC SQUAMOUS CELL CARCINOMA OF THE ANAL CANAL WITH CYTOTOXIC CHEMOTHERAPY

Because SCCA represents an uncommon GI malignancy for which a small fraction of patients will develop distant metastases, the role of systemic chemotherapy in the management of metastatic disease remains an understudied topic for which extensive experience and robust data are lacking. Indeed, no prospective trial for metastatic SCCA using cytotoxic chemotherapeutic agents has ever been completed. At present, there is no accepted standard of care consensus for the management of distant disease. At large academic referral centers, the treatment approach is based upon published work in the literature from case series and small respective cohorts.

The combination of cisplatin and 5-fluorouracil has been reported as efficacious in multiple small series, and this chemotherapy doublet is the lone recommended therapy for the treatment of metastatic disease by the National Comprehensive Cancer Network (NCCN) panel. One initial report utilizing this combination involved 3 patients at a single institution with metastatic SCCA involving the liver.[40] All patients here demonstrated partial or complete radiographic responses to this regimen, with 2 of the 3 patients experiencing drastic reductions in their tumor volumes, which led to prolonged survival outcomes. This series, however, included patients who had liver involvement as the only site of distant metastases. Nonetheless, it did provide some optimism regarding the use of cisplatin and 5-fluorouracil in the management of metastatic SCCA, consistent with known understanding that these agents have activity in the treatment of advanced/unresectable squamous cell cancers of other primary sites as well. Another single-institution series of 19 patients with metastatic SCCA who had involvement of many different sites of distant metastases examined the use of cisplatin with 5-fluorouracil.[41] Here, 1 complete response was observed, and there were 11 partial responses (response rate 66%). The most common grade 3 to 4 toxicities were noted to be nausea (30%) and nonfebrile neutropenia (13%). At 1 year following initiation of treatment, 62% of patients were still alive, and 32% remained alive at 5 years, for a median survival of 34.5 months. Although the numbers of patients for both of these series are small, they do provide some suggestion that the use of cisplatin with 5-fluorouracil is active and associated with a tolerable toxicity profile for patients with metastatic SCCA.

With a lack of available options for treatment of distant metastases, other groups examined the role of taxanes as a therapeutic approach for the treatment of metastatic SCCA. The combination of carboplatin with paclitaxel is approved for the use of other advanced squamous cell tumors. One single-institution series recently reported outcomes of 18 patients with metastatic SCCA treated with this regimen.[42] Here, 12 patients were administered this doublet as the first-line treatment for their metastatic disease. Radiographic responses were noted in 53% of patients, with 3 complete responses detected. Grade 3 to 4 toxicities were noted in 6 of 18 patients, with the most common toxicity being neutropenia (N = 4). Median overall survival in this cohort was approximately 12 months.

Other series have examined the use of paclitaxel as a single agent following progression on frontline cisplatin/5-fluorouracil. One report detailed the use of paclitaxel at a dose of 175 mg/m^2 every 3 weeks in 5 patients, 2 of whom were noted to be HIV-positive.[43] Disease control (defined as either radiographic response or stable disease) was observed in 3 of these 5 patients. In a separate report of 7 patients with metastatic SCCA who were treated with single-agent paclitaxel at a single institution, partial responses were observed in 4 patients, and stable disease was observed in 1 additional patient.[44] Again, the role of taxanes in the management of metastatic SCCA, whether with or without carboplatin, remains unclear at present. These series should be interpreted with caution given the small number of patients who were included in the analyses.

Integrating both of these approaches, other small cohorts reported results for patients with metastatic SCCA using a triple combination of paclitaxel, carboplatin, and 5-fluorouracil. A prospective phase II trial of these 3 agents for patients with advanced squamous cell cancers of multiple primary sites included 7 patients with metastatic anal cancer. Four patients had radiographic responses, 2 of which were complete radiographic responses.[45] A different series of 8 patients with metastatic SCCA treated with the same 3 cytotoxic chemotherapeutic agents revealed complete responses in 4 patients and progressive disease in the remaining patients.[46] Overall, these 8 patients demonstrated acceptable toxicity from the triple combination of docetaxel, cisplatin, and 5-fluorouracil.

To date, the largest retrospective series for metastatic SCCA percent was reported from cohort of patients treated at M.D. Anderson.[47] Here, 77 patients were examined, with 42 patients (55%) administered 5-fluorouracil/cisplatin, and 24 patients (31%) receiving carboplatin/paclitaxel. Response rates were nominally better with 5-fluorouracil/cisplatin (57%) relative to carboplatin/paclitaxel (33%), although no definitive conclusions can be made from these findings given their noncontrolled and retrospective nature.

As there is no accepted standard of care for the treatment in the front-line setting of metastatic SCCA, a prospective International Rare Cancer Initiative (IRCI)/Eastern Cooperative Oncology Group (ECOG) - American College of Radiology Imaging Network (ACRIN) randomized, phase II trial (EA2133/InterACCT) is ongoing to compare the combinations of cisplatin/5-fluorouracil and carboplatin/paclitaxel for patients with SCCA who have never received any prior systemic chemotherapy for distant metastatic disease. The primary end point for this study is response rate, and the goal is to identify the best chemotherapeutic backbone upon which additional biologic and/or immunotherapeutic agents can be added in future studies, with the goal of improving survival outcomes for patients with metastatic SCCA.

ROLE OF BIOLOGIC AGENTS IN THE TREATMENT OF METASTATIC SQUAMOUS CELL CARCINOMA OF THE ANAL CANAL

To date, the use of targeted therapies in the management of metastatic SCCA has been limited by a lack of understanding regarding the genomic profiling patterns that drive tumor development. Despite mutations in KRAS and NRAS being prevalent in tumors arising from the adjacent colorectum,[48–51] multiple series analyzing anal tumors have failed to detect RAS mutations in SCCA.[52–54] In addition, anal tumors have been frequently reported to express epidermal growth factor receptor (EGFR) at high levels on the surface of the cancer cell.[55] Based on these findings, multiple series have examined the role of anti-EGFR monoclonal antibodies like cetuximab, which targets EGFR signaling extracellularly.

One series from M.D. Anderson reported results from 17 patients who received cetuximab, either as a single agent or in combination with systemic chemotherapy, following progression on at least 1 prior line of systemic therapy for metastatic disease.[56] Radiographic responses were noted in 6 of 17 patients (response rate 35%), and anti–EGFR therapy was overall well tolerated in this group of patients. Another group reported outcomes of 5 patients with a RAS wild-type metastatic SCCA who received cetuximab with or without irinotecan.[57] Partial responses were noted in 3 of these patients. These results provide optimism that anti–EGFR therapy can be utilized safely in the management of metastatic SCCA. However, to date, no prospective trials comparing cytotoxic chemotherapy with or without anti-EGFR therapy have been performed, and so the added benefit of agents like cetuximab in this setting remains unclear.

Vascular endothelial growth factor (VEGF) is an important mediator for angiogenesis in the development of new tumors.[58] Bevacizumab is a monoclonal antibody that targets VEGF.[59] Recent results of a large prospective trial in patients with metastatic cervical cancer, another solid tumor strongly associated with coinfection by HPV, compared traditional cytotoxic chemotherapy regimens with or without bevacizumab.[60] Strikingly, patients with advanced cervical cancer who received chemotherapy in combination with bevacizumab demonstrated improved overall survival as well as higher response rates to treatment. This drug also has activity as monotherapy for patients with metastatic cancer of the cervix.[61] Together, these results provide important rationale toward extension of these findings to the management of metastatic anal cancer. Further studies are warranted to investigate the role of anti-VEGF therapies in incurable SCCA.

ROLE OF SURGERY AND RADIATION IN THE MANAGEMENT OF DISTANT METASTASES

In the previously mentioned retrospective series of 77 patients at M.D. Anderson with metastatic SCCA, 2 distinct cohorts of patients were noted: patients with oligometastatic disease amenable to multimodality therapy and patients with diffuse, disseminated disease who were candidates for systemic chemotherapy only.[47] Here, 33 patients had oligometastatic disease that was amenable to locoregional therapy, 19 with surgical resection and 14 with chemoradiation to their limited sites of distant metastases. The most frequent sites of surgical resection included liver, lung, and distant lymph nodes. Comparison of patients with metastatic SCCA here who were and were not able to proceed toward surgery and/or chemoradiation for distant tumor involvement revealed a strong survival benefit for those patients who were able to receive multidisciplinary treatment (53 months vs 17 months, $P<.001$). Importantly, these findings suggest heterogeneity within the population of patients with metastatic SCCA and that identifying patients with oligometastatic disease who may be amenable to surgery and/or chemoradiation is important given the possibility of improving survival outcomes with treatment approaches other than systemic chemotherapy. The authors recommend referral of such patients to major academic centers with extensive experience in the treatment of metastatic SCCA for evaluation of multimodality therapy.

THE ROLE OF IMMUNOTHERAPY IN THE MANAGEMENT OF METASTATIC SQUAMOUS CELL CARCINOMA OF THE ANAL CANAL

In recent years, multiple prospective trials have reported profound clinical responses and prolonged survival with the use of immune checkpoint blockade agents in advanced/metastatic diseases such as melanoma, nonsmall cell lung cancer, renal cell carcinoma, and Hodgkin lymphoma.[62–68] These agents target proteins like PD–1 and CTLA–4 on the surface of immune cells in the tumor microenvironment, which, upon binding to their respective ligands on the surface of adjacent tumor cells, function to down-regulate the effector cytotoxic T-cell response against the tumor cell and promote tumor cell evasion from an immune attack.[69–74]

Given the strong association between prior infection with HPV and the development of SCCA, it is reasonable that these tumors would be immunogenic and thereby susceptible to recognition of an immune response. Indeed, the HPV viral oncoproteins E6 and E7 can be detected by antigen-presenting cells and recruit tumor infiltrating lymphocytes into the adjacent tumor microenvironment to create a more inflamed tumor.[75–77]

Nivolumab and pembrolizumab are monoclonal antibodies against PD–1. Recently, a phase Ib trial of 25 patients with metastatic anal cancer who were treated with pembrolizumab was reported.[78] Eighty-eight percent of patients had squamous cell cancers, although there were patients with carcinoid, endometrioid, and mucoendometrioid cancers who were treated on study. PD–L1 expression by immunohistochemistry was required for participation. Overall, pembrolizumab was tolerated well with an acceptable toxicity profile, with nausea, fatigue, and diarrhea being the most common adverse events reported. Radiographic responses by Response Evaluation Criteria in Solid Tumors (RECIST) 1.1 criteria were observed in 5 of 25 patients (response rate 20%). Definitive conclusions cannot be drawn at this point from these results given that the population of anal cancer histologies allowed was heterogeneous and also because this study was not designed to test efficacy normally.

However, the prospective NCI 9673 phase II trial of nivolumab as a single agent for patients with metastatic SCCA who had progressed on at least 1 prior line of chemotherapy for distant disease completed enrollment, and early results were recently reported.[79] Unlike the previous study with pembrolizumab, NCI 9673 was designed with the primary end point to measure response rate with treatment using single-agent nivolumab. Here, 37 patients with metastatic SCCA were treated at multiple sites across the United States. Among 34 patients who were available for response, 2 complete responses were observed, and 7 additional patients had partial radiographic responses by RECIST 1.1 criteria (response rate 26%). Grade 3 adverse events were reported in 5 patients and included anemia, rash, fatigue, and immune-mediated hypothyroidism. This trial also allowed HIV-positive patients to participate provided that their CD4 count exceeded 300 cells/mm^3. This trial was the first prospective clinical study ever to be completed for patients with metastatic SCCA who had progressed on prior systemic chemotherapy for distant metastases. The final analyses for this trial have not yet been reported but are eagerly anticipated. Nonetheless, given the unmet need for this patient population, that nivolumab demonstrated both safety/tolerability and efficacy generates optimism for introducing novel immunotherapy approaches into the clinics as a means to improve survival outcomes for this patient population. An extension of the NCI 9673 study to combined nivolumab with ipilimumab, a monoclonal antibody against CTLA-4, is currently being planned, as this combination of immunotherapy checkpoint blockade agents has demonstrated even further survival benefit in other immunogenic advanced solid tumors.

REFERENCES

1. Siegel RL, Miller KD, Jemal A. Cancer statistics, 2016. CA Cancer J Clin 2016; 66(1):7–30.
2. Schiller DE, Cummings BJ, Rai S, et al. Outcomes of salvage surgery for squamous cell carcinoma of the anal canal. Ann Surg Oncol 2007;14(10):2780–9.
3. Das P, Bhatia S, Eng C, et al. Predictors and patterns of recurrence after definitive chemoradiation for anal cancer. Int J Radiat Oncol Biol Phys 2007;68(3):794–800.
4. Cummings BJ. Metastatic anal cancer: the search for cure. Onkologie 2006; 29(1–2):5–6.
5. Johnson LG, Madeleine MM, Newcomer LM, et al. Anal cancer incidence and survival: the surveillance, epidemiology, and end results experience, 1973–2000. Cancer 2004;101(2):281–8.
6. Frisch M, Glimelius B, van den Brule AJ, et al. Sexually transmitted infection as a cause of anal cancer. N Engl J Med 1997;337(19):1350–8.
7. Daling JR, Madeleine MM, Johnson LG, et al. Human papillomavirus, smoking, and sexual practices in the etiology of anal cancer. Cancer 2004;101(2): 270–80.
8. Frisch M, Biggar RJ, Goedert JJ. Human papillomavirus-associated cancers in patients with human immunodeficiency virus infection and acquired immunodeficiency syndrome. J Natl Cancer Inst 2000;92(18):1500–10.

9. Sunesen KG, Norgaard M, Thorlacius-Ussing O, et al. Immunosuppressive disorders and risk of anal squamous cell carcinoma: a nationwide cohort study in Denmark, 1978-2005. Int J Cancer 2010;127(3):675–84.

10. Ryan DP, Compton CC, Mayer RJ. Carcinoma of the anal canal. N Engl J Med 2000;342(11):792–800.

11. De Vuyst H, Clifford GM, Nascimento MC, et al. Prevalence and type distribution of human papillomavirus in carcinoma and intraepithelial neoplasia of the vulva, vagina and anus: a meta-analysis. Int J Cancer 2009;124(7):1626–36.

12. Hoots BE, Palefsky JM, Pimenta JM, et al. Human papillomavirus type distribution in anal cancer and anal intraepithelial lesions. Int J Cancer 2009;124(10): 2375–83.

13. Kjaer SK, Frederiksen K, Munk C, et al. Long-term absolute risk of cervical intraepithelial neoplasia grade 3 or worse following human papillomavirus infection: role of persistence. J Natl Cancer Inst 2010;102(19):1478–88.

14. Rodriguez AC, Schiffman M, Herrero R, et al. Longitudinal study of human papillomavirus persistence and cervical intraepithelial neoplasia grade 2/3: critical role of duration of infection. J Natl Cancer Inst 2010;102(5):315–24.

15. Gillison ML, Koch WM, Capone RB, et al. Evidence for a causal association between human papillomavirus and a subset of head and neck cancers. J Natl Cancer Inst 2000;92(9):709–20.

16. D'Souza G, Kreimer AR, Viscidi R, et al. Case–control study of human papillomavirus and oropharyngeal cancer. N Engl J Med 2007;356(19):1944–56.

17. Sturgis EM, Cinciripini PM. Trends in head and neck cancer incidence in relation to smoking prevalence: an emerging epidemic of human papillomavirus-associated cancers? Cancer 2007;110(7):1429–35.

18. Daling JR, Madeleine MM, Johnson LG, et al. Penile cancer: importance of circumcision, human papillomavirus and smoking in in situ and invasive disease. Int J Cancer 2005;116(4):606–16.

19. Sarkar FH, Miles BJ, Plieth DH, et al. Detection of human papillomavirus in squamous neoplasm of the penis. J Urol 1992;147(2):389–92.

20. Gargano JW, Wilkinson EJ, Unger ER, et al. Prevalence of human papillomavirus types in invasive vulvar cancers and vulvar intraepithelial neoplasia 3 in the United States before vaccine introduction. J Low Genit Tract Dis 2012;16(4): 471–9.

21. Werness BA, Levine AJ, Howley PM. Association of human papillomavirus types 16 and 18 E6 proteins with p53. Science 1990;248(4951):76–9.

22. Li X, Coffino P. High-risk human papillomavirus E6 protein has two distinct binding sites within p53, of which only one determines degradation. J Virol 1996; 70(7):4509–16.

23. Balsitis SJ, Sage J, Duensing S, et al. Recapitulation of the effects of the human papillomavirus type 16 E7 oncogene on mouse epithelium by somatic Rb deletion and detection of pRb-independent effects of E7 in vivo. Mol Cell Biol 2003;23(24): 9094–103.

24. Morris VK, Rashid A, Rodriguez-Bigas M, et al. Clinicopathologic features associated with human papillomavirus/p16 in patients with metastatic squamous cell carcinoma of the anal canal. Oncologist 2015;20(11):1247–52.

25. Serup-Hansen E, Linnemann D, Skovrider-Ruminski W, et al. Human papillomavirus genotyping and p16 expression as prognostic factors for patients with American Joint Committee on Cancer stages I to III carcinoma of the anal canal. J Clin Oncol 2014;32(17):1812–7.

26. Mai S, Welzel G, Ottstadt M, et al. Prognostic Relevance of HPV Infection and p16 overexpression in squamous cell anal cancer. Int J Radiat Oncol Biol Phys 2015; 93(4):819–27.

27. Baricevic I, He X, Chakrabarty B, et al. High-sensitivity human papilloma virus genotyping reveals near universal positivity in anal squamous cell carcinoma: different implications for vaccine prevention and prognosis. Eur J Cancer 2015; 51(6):776–85.

28. FUTURE II Study Group. Quadrivalent vaccine against human papillomavirus to prevent high-grade cervical lesions. N Engl J Med 2007;356(19):1915–27.

29. Joura EA, Giuliano AR, Iversen OE, et al. A 9-valent HPV vaccine against infection and intraepithelial neoplasia in women. N Engl J Med 2015;372(8):711–23.

30. Palefsky JM, Giuliano AR, Goldstone S, et al. HPV vaccine against anal HPV infection and anal intraepithelial neoplasia. N Engl J Med 2011;365(17):1576–85.

31. Nigro ND, Vaitkevicius VK, Considine B Jr. Combined therapy for cancer of the anal canal: a preliminary report. Dis Colon Rectum 1974;17(3):354–6.

32. Cummings BJ, Keane TJ, O'Sullivan B, et al. Epidermoid anal cancer: treatment by radiation alone or by radiation and 5-fluorouracil with and without mitomycin C. Int J Radiat Oncol Biol Phys 1991;21(5):1115–25.

33. Ajani JA, Winter KA, Gunderson LL, et al. Fluorouracil, mitomycin, and radiotherapy vs fluorouracil, cisplatin, and radiotherapy for carcinoma of the anal canal: a randomized controlled trial. JAMA 2008;299(16):1914–21.

34. James RD, Glynne-Jones R, Meadows HM, et al. Mitomycin or cisplatin chemoradiation with or without maintenance chemotherapy for treatment of squamous-cell carcinoma of the anus (ACT II): a randomised, phase 3, open-label, 2 x 2 factorial trial. Lancet Oncol 2013;14(6):516–24.

35. Gunderson LL, Winter KA, Ajani JA, et al. Long-term update of US GI intergroup RTOG 98-11 phase III trial for anal carcinoma: survival, relapse, and colostomy failure with concurrent chemoradiation involving fluorouracil/mitomycin versus fluorouracil/cisplatin. J Clin Oncol 2012;30(35):4344–51.

36. Mullen JT, Rodriguez-Bigas MA, Chang GJ, et al. Results of surgical salvage after failed chemoradiation therapy for epidermoid carcinoma of the anal canal. Ann Surg Oncol 2007;14(2):478–83.

37. Allal AS, Laurencet FM, Reymond MA, et al. Effectiveness of surgical salvage therapy for patients with locally uncontrolled anal carcinoma after sphincter-conserving treatment. Cancer 1999;86(3):405–9.

38. Ellenhorn JD, Enker WE, Quan SH. Salvage abdominoperineal resection following combined chemotherapy and radiotherapy for epidermoid carcinoma of the anus. Ann Surg Oncol 1994;1(2):105–10.

39. Nilsson PJ, Svensson C, Goldman S, et al. Salvage abdominoperineal resection in anal epidermoid cancer. Br J Surg 2002;89(11):1425–9.

40. Ajani JA, Carrasco CH, Jackson DE, et al. Combination of cisplatin plus fluoropyrimidine chemotherapy effective against liver metastases from carcinoma of the anal canal. Am J Med 1989;87(2):221–4.

41. Faivre C, Rougier P, Ducreux M, et al. 5-fluorouracile and cisplatinum combination chemotherapy for metastatic squamous-cell anal cancer. Bull Cancer 1999;86(10):861–5 [in French].

42. Kim R, Byer J, Fulp WJ, et al. Carboplatin and paclitaxel treatment is effective in advanced anal cancer. Oncology 2014;87(2):125–32.

43. Alcindor T. Activity of paclitaxel in metastatic squamous anal carcinoma. Int J Colorectal Dis 2008;23(7):717.

44. Abbas A, Nehme E, Fakih M. Single-agent paclitaxel in advanced anal cancer after failure of cisplatin and 5-fluorouracil chemotherapy. Anticancer Res 2011; 31(12):4637–40.
45. Hainsworth JD, Burris HA 3rd, Meluch AA, et al. Paclitaxel, carboplatin, and long-term continuous infusion of 5-fluorouracil in the treatment of advanced squamous and other selected carcinomas: results of a phase II trial. Cancer 2001;92(3): 642–9.
46. Kim S, Jary M, Mansi L, et al. DCF (docetaxel, cisplatin and 5-fluorouracil) chemotherapy is a promising treatment for recurrent advanced squamous cell anal carcinoma. Ann Oncol 2013;24(12):3045–50.
47. Eng C, Chang GJ, You YN, et al. The role of systemic chemotherapy and multi-disciplinary management in improving the overall survival of patients with meta-static squamous cell carcinoma of the anal canal. Oncotarget 2014;5(22): 11133–42.
48. Cancer Genome Atlas Network. Comprehensive molecular characterization of human colon and rectal cancer. Nature 2012;487(7407):330–7.
49. Price TJ, Bruhn MA, Lee CK, et al. Correlation of extended RAS and PIK3CA gene mutation status with outcomes from the phase III AGITG MAX study involving capecitabine alone or in combination with bevacizumab plus or minus mitomycin C in advanced colorectal cancer. Br J Cancer 2015;112(6):963–70.
50. Roth AD, Tejpar S, Delorenzi M, et al. Prognostic role of KRAS and BRAF in stage II and III resected colon cancer: results of the translational study on the PETACC-3, EORTC 40993, SAKK 60-00 trial. J Clin Oncol 2010;28(3):466–74.
51. Amado RG, Wolf M, Peeters M, et al. Wild-type KRAS is required for panitumumab efficacy in patients with metastatic colorectal cancer. J Clin Oncol 2008; 26(10):1626–34.
52. Serup-Hansen E, Linnemann D, Hogdall E, et al. KRAS and BRAF mutations in anal carcinoma. APMIS 2015;123(1):53–9.
53. Chung JH, Sanford E, Johnson A, et al. Comprehensive genomic profiling of anal squamous cell carcinoma reveals distinct genomically defined classes. Ann Oncol 2016;27(7):1336–41.
54. Smaglo BG, Tesfaye A, Halfdanarson TR, et al. Comprehensive multiplatform biomarker analysis of 199 anal squamous cell carcinomas. Oncotarget 2015; 6(41):43594–604.
55. Le LH, Chetty R, Moore MJ. Epidermal growth factor receptor expression in anal canal carcinoma. Am J Clin Pathol 2005;124(1):20–3.
56. Rogers JE, Ohinata A, Silva NN, et al. Epidermal growth factor receptor inhibition in metastatic anal cancer. Anticancer Drugs 2016;27:804–8.
57. Lukan N, Strobel P, Willer A, et al. Cetuximab-based treatment of metastatic anal cancer: correlation of response with KRAS mutational status. Oncology 2009; 77(5):293–9.
58. Leung DW, Cachianes G, Kuang WJ, et al. Vascular endothelial growth factor is a secreted angiogenic mitogen. Science 1989;246(4935):1306–9.
59. Ferrara N, Hillan KJ, Gerber HP, et al. Discovery and development of bevacizumab, an anti-VEGF antibody for treating cancer. Nat Rev Drug Discov 2004; 3(5):391–400.
60. Tewari KS, Sill MW, Long HJ 3rd, et al. Improved survival with bevacizumab in advanced cervical cancer. N Engl J Med 2014;370(8):734–43.
61. Monk BJ, Sill MW, Burger RA, et al. Phase II trial of bevacizumab in the treatment of persistent or recurrent squamous cell carcinoma of the cervix: a gynecologic oncology group study. J Clin Oncol 2009;27(7):1069–74.

62. Postow MA, Chesney J, Pavlick AC, et al. Nivolumab and ipilimumab versus ipilimumab in untreated melanoma. N Engl J Med 2015;372(21):2006–17.
63. Larkin J, Chiarion-Sileni V, Gonzalez R, et al. Combined nivolumab and ipilimumab or monotherapy in untreated melanoma. N Engl J Med 2015;373(1):23–34.
64. Hodi FS, O'Day SJ, McDermott DF, et al. Improved survival with ipilimumab in patients with metastatic melanoma. N Engl J Med 2010;363(8):711–23.
65. Topalian SL, Hodi FS, Brahmer JR, et al. Safety, activity, and immune correlates of anti-PD-1 antibody in cancer. N Engl J Med 2012;366(26):2443–54.
66. Ansell SM, Lesokhin AM, Borrello I, et al. PD-1 blockade with nivolumab in relapsed or refractory Hodgkin's lymphoma. N Engl J Med 2015;372(4):311–9.
67. Motzer RJ, Escudier B, McDermott DF, et al. Nivolumab versus everolimus in advanced renal-cell carcinoma. N Engl J Med 2015;373(19):1803–13.
68. Brahmer J, Reckamp KL, Baas P, et al. Nivolumab versus docetaxel in advanced squamous-cell non-small-cell lung cancer. N Engl J Med 2015;373(2):123–35.
69. Ishida Y, Agata Y, Shibahara K, et al. Induced expression of PD-1, a novel member of the immunoglobulin gene superfamily, upon programmed cell death. EMBO J 1992;11(11):3887–95.
70. Schneider H, Downey J, Smith A, et al. Reversal of the TCR stop signal by CTLA-4. Science 2006;313(5795):1972–5.
71. Qureshi OS, Zheng Y, Nakamura K, et al. Trans-endocytosis of CD80 and CD86: a molecular basis for the cell-extrinsic function of CTLA-4. Science 2011; 332(6029):600–3.
72. Krummel MF, Allison JP. CTLA-4 engagement inhibits IL-2 accumulation and cell cycle progression upon activation of resting T cells. J Exp Med 1996;183(6):2533–40.
73. Freeman GJ, Long AJ, Iwai Y, et al. Engagement of the PD-1 immunoinhibitory receptor by a novel B7 family member leads to negative regulation of lymphocyte activation. J Exp Med 2000;192(7):1027–34.
74. Keir ME, Liang SC, Guleria I, et al. Tissue expression of PD-L1 mediates peripheral T cell tolerance. J Exp Med 2006;203(4):883–95.
75. de Jong A, van der Burg SH, Kwappenberg KM, et al. Frequent detection of human papillomavirus 16 E2-specific T-helper immunity in healthy subjects. Cancer Res 2002;62(2):472–9.
76. de Jong A, van Poelgeest MI, van der Hulst JM, et al. Human papillomavirus type 16-positive cervical cancer is associated with impaired CD4+ T-cell immunity against early antigens E2 and E6. Cancer Res 2004;64(15):5449–55.
77. Welters MJ, de Jong A, van den Eeden SJ, et al. Frequent display of human papillomavirus type 16 E6-specific memory t-Helper cells in the healthy population as witness of previous viral encounter. Cancer Res 2003;63(3):636–41.
78. Ott PA, Piha-Paul SA, Munster P, et al. Pembrolizumab (MK-3475) for PD-L1-positive squamous cell carcinoma (SCC) of the anal canal: preliminary safety and efficacy results from KEYNOTE-028. Paper presented at: European Cancer Congress, Vienna, September 26, 2015.
79. Morris VK II, Ciombor KK, Salem ME, et al. NCI9673: a multi-institutional eETCTN phase II study of nivolumab in refractory metastatic squamous cell carcinoma of the anal canal (SCCA). Presented at: American Society of Clinical Oncology. Chicago, June 5, 2016.

Uncommon Anal Neoplasms

Amitesh C. Roy, MD, MSc, FRACP[a,b], David Wattchow, BM BS, PhD, FRACS[b,c],
David Astill, BSc Hons, BMBS, PhD, FRCPA[b,d], Simron Singh, BSc, MD, MPH, FRCPC[e,f],
Susan Pendlebury, MBBS, FRANZCR[g], Kirsten Gormly, MBBS, FRANZCR[h],
Eva Segelov, MBBS, PhD, FRACP[i,*]

KEYWORDS

- Unusual cancers • Anal neuroendocrine tumor • Anal melanoma • Anal lymphoma

KEY POINTS

- Unusual cases of anal cancer comprise histologies of anal gland and canal adenocarcinoma, anal lymphoma, anal neuroendocrine tumors, and anal melanomas.
- Incidence is likely to rise with the greater use of colonoscopy and better imaging techniques, such as MRI.
- Management is based on usual treatment of underlying tumor type rather than that of anal epithelioid cancer.
- Improvements in outcome may result from an effort to collect rare cases of anal cancer on an international database.

Anal cancer is a rare disease with epidermoid cancers accounting for 1% to 2% of all digestive tract malignancies.[1] Less common anal neoplasms comprise approximately 20% to 25% of these,[2] including anal canal adenocarcinoma, anorectal melanoma, mesenchymal and neurogenic tumors of the anal canal (in particular gastrointestinal

The authors have nothing to disclose.
[a] Department of Medical Oncology, Flinders Centre for Innovation in Cancer, Flinders Medical Centre, Flinders Drive Bedford Park, South Australia, 5042 Australia; [b] Department of Surgery, Flinders University, Sturt Road, Bedford Park, South Australia 5042, Australia; [c] Department of Surgery, Flinders Medical Centre, Flinders Drive Bedford Park, South Australia, 5042, Australia; [d] Department of Anatomical Pathology, SA Pathology (Flinders Medical Centre), Flinders Drive Bedford Park, South Australia 5042, Australia; [e] Division of Medical Oncology, Odette Cancer Centre, Sunnybrook Health Sciences Centre, 2075 Bayview Ave, Toronto, ON M4N 3M5, Canada Toronto, Ontario, Canada; [f] Department of Medicine, Medical Sciences Building, 1 King's College Cir #3172, University of Toronto, Toronto, ON M5S 1A8, Canada; [g] Department of Radiation Oncology, St Vincent's Hospital, Victoria Street, Darlinghurst, Sydney, 2010 New South Wales, Australia; [h] Department of Radiology, Dr Jones & Partners Medical Imaging, Tennyson Centre, 520 South Road, Kurralta Park South Australia 5037, Australia; [i] Department of Medicine, St Vincent's Clinical School, St Vincent's Hospital, University of New South Wales, Level 5 de Lacy, 438 Victoria Street, Darlinghurst, Sydney, New South Wales 2010, Australia
* Corresponding author.
E-mail address: e.segelov@unsw.edu.au

stromal tumors [GIST], schwannomas, and sarcomas), neuroendocrine tumors (NETs), lymphoma, and basal cell carcinoma (BCC). The anal canal is also a rare site for metastasis from other primary malignancies. As imaging technology improves, particularly MRI, and colonoscopy becomes routine, many rarer tumors are detected incidentally. Diligent linkage of clinical features with expert histopathology assessment identifies uncommon anal neoplasms to ensure that appropriate management is instituted.

ADENOCARCINOMA OF THE ANAL CANAL

Adenocarcinoma of the anal canal (ACA) accounts for 5% to 19% of all anal canal cancers.[3,4] These are subclassified under the World Health Organization Classification of Tumors into three main subtypes: (1) colorectal-type adenocarcinoma, (2) anal gland adenocarcinoma, and (3) fistula-associated adenocarcinoma.[5] In addition, a form of intraepithelial adenocarcinoma, also known as Paget disease, is a distinct entity and affects areas with a high density of apocrine glands around the anogenital region.

The clinical signs of adenocarcinoma, such as anal squamous cell anal cancer (SCC), are often nonspecific and the diagnosis is commonly made serendipitously in patients undergoing excision of presumed benign conditions. Management of ACA is challenging because of its rarity, difficulty in confirming diagnosis, and lack of direct evidence for particular clinical management strategies.[6] There is little information regarding risk factors; however, there is some linkage to high-risk subtypes of human papilloma virus, mainly subtype 18.[7]

Colorectal-Type Adenocarcinoma

These tumors represent either downward spread of a primary rectal adenocarcinoma (RA) or de novo carcinoma arising in residual glandular cells of the anal transition zone just above the dentate line. In contrast to a rectal-based adenocarcinoma, there is a higher risk of inguinal and femoral nodal involvement because of the dual lymphatic drainage of the anus.[8] Histologically and clinically these cancers are indistinguishable from usual rectal tumors and apart from their anatomic location do not represent a special entity. In most cases the histologic diagnosis is straightforward. However, on immunohistochemistry, colorectal-type ACA may have unexpected cytokeratin (CK) 7 expression, although this is usually accompanied by coexpression of CK20.[6] This is different from anal gland carcinomas, which usually are CK20 negative.

In practice, tumors used to be classified as rectal cancers on digital examination if their epicenter was located greater than 2 cm proximal to the dentate line or the anorectal ring, and as anal canal cancers if their epicenter was less than 2 cm below the dentate line.[9] Newer imaging techniques, such as MRI, assist with delineating site of origin more accurately, particularly if there is a polypoid stalk (**Figs. 1** and **2**).

Anal Gland Adenocarcinoma

Anal gland tumors usually originate from the anal ducts and demonstrate continuity with the anal gland epithelium. There are only a few case reports demonstrating convincing evidence of the origin of the tumor from an anal gland.[10–13] These tumors are sometimes termed as "anal duct adenocarcinoma" because of their putative origin and are characterized histologically by the combination of ductal and mucinous areas. Hobbs and colleagues[14] defined the following criteria: cells haphazardly dispersed, invading the wall of the anorectal area, containing small glands with little mucin production and without an intraluminal component; and immune-histochemical positivity for CK7. Kuroda and colleagues[15] have demonstrated that CK7, CK19, and MUC5AC immune-histochemical reactivity is a marker for adenocarcinoma of anal gland origin.

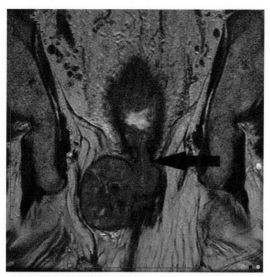

Fig. 1. MRI coronal T2-weighted: polypoidal adenocarcinoma (*arrow*) from low rectum.

In clinical practice, if tumor is present within the anal canal wall, without a pre-existing fistula or dysplasia of the surface mucosa, then irrespective of the extent of mucin production it is more likely to be anal gland adenocarcinoma.

Adenocarcinoma Within Anorectal Fistula

Anorectal fistulae may be developmental or acquired secondary to underlying inflammatory bowel disease, such as Crohn disease.[16–18] Adenocarcinomas arising in anorectal fistulae usually have the histologic appearance of a well-differentiated mucinous adenocarcinoma; however, tubular adenocarcinomas and squamous cell neoplasia can also be present[17,19,20] (**Fig. 3**). The cell of origin could be related to either rectal-type glandular mucosa or anal glands or ducts. Occasionally there is evidence of epithelioid granulomas secondary to inflammation or extravasated mucin, in the absence of other signs of underlying inflammatory bowel disease. Rarely, adenocarcinomas can arise in congenital duplications of the lower part of the hindgut, which can be lined by rectal mucosa that has a tendency to become malignant.[17]

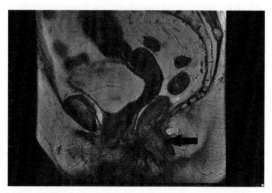

Fig. 2. MRI sagittal T2-weighted: anal canal adenocarcinoma (*arrow*).

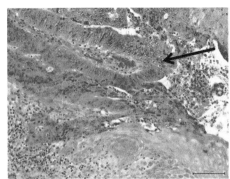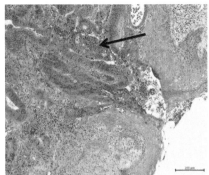

Fig. 3. Adenocarcinoma of the anal canal. Malignant glands (*arrows*) are seen extending from the luminal surface, underrunning the adjacent squamous epithelium and infiltrating the surrounding soft tissues.

Management of Anal Adenocarcinoma

Locoregional disease

Importantly, the management of adenocarcinomas arising in the anal canal follows the same principles as rectal cancer, rather than SCC anus. The primary treatment is surgical resection, typically abdominoperineal resection (APR) because sphincter preservation is not achievable. The literature supports surgical resection as providing the lowest rates of local relapse, recognizing that with historical data sets there is inevitable selection bias. Based on limited data, survival rates seem to be improved with multimodality management with chemotherapy and radiotherapy given before or after surgery, with improvement in local and systemic control.[2,3,8,10,21] For anal adenocarcinoma, data exist for benefit from radiation therapy given either neoadjuvantly or adjuvantly for T3-4 and N1-2 stage, as per rectal cancer.[22,23] Intensity modulated radiation therapy (IMRT) and Volumetric modulated arc therapy (VMAT) techniques are recommended and treatment volume should reflect the lymphatic drainage of the anus, including inguinal lymph nodes.[23]

Prognosis

Only limited case series have been reported. The most recent data from a Surveillance, Epidemiology and End Results database review from 1990 to 2011 compared survival of patients diagnosed with ACA, anal SCC, and RA. Median overall survival (OS) of patients with ACA was 33 months, compared with SCC of 118 months and RA of 68 months ($P<.01$). Multivariate analysis demonstrated that ACA had worse prognosis than SCC (hazard ratio, 0.66; 95% confidence interval, 0.59–0.75; $P<.01$) and RA (hazard ratio, 0.68; 95% confidence interval, 0.61–0.77; $P<.01$). Improved survival was observed in patients who underwent radical surgery (hazard ratio, 0.71; 95% confidence interval, 0.51–1.00; $P = .05$).[4]

The importance of resection of adenocarcinomas arising in the anal canal was demonstrated in a retrospective series from MD Anderson Cancer Center in which 16 patients were treated between 1976 and 1998 with either primary radiotherapy or definitive chemoradiation (no surgery).[22] When compared stage for stage with 92 patients with SCC treated with definitive chemoradiation, patients with ACA had a higher 5-year local recurrence rate (18% for SCC vs 54% for ACA) and worse disease-free survival (DFS) (77% vs 19%, respectively) and 5-year OS (85% vs 64%).

A multicenter retrospective study (1974–2000) from the Rare Cancer Network compared 82 patients treated with different modalities. The 5-year actuarial local relapse rate was 20% for APR (n = 6), 37% for radiotherapy plus surgery (n = 45), and 36% for definitive chemoradiation (n = 31). The 5-year OS was 21%, 29%, and 58%, respectively; 5-year DFS was 22%, 25%, and 54%.[23] Such data support the role of radiotherapy and raise the potential of definitive chemoradiation allowing sphincter preservation.

Metastatic disease

As with local therapy, management of metastatic disease follows the protocols used for colorectal cancer. Combination or single-agent palliative chemotherapy is used to prolong survival and improve local control and quality of life (QoL). There is paucity of data informing the choice of chemotherapy regimens or the role of newer targeted drugs. Overall outcome seems to be worse than patients with metastatic colorectal cancer.[24]

PAGET DISEASE OF THE ANAL CANAL

Paget disease of anal canal falls under the extramammary Paget disease group and was first described by Crocker[25] in 1889. It most commonly occurs in elderly patients and manifests as red or white-crusted patches of skin with associated pruritus in the anal region. Paget disease can also occur in other anogenital sites, most commonly in vulval skin, perineum, and anal margin skin. Primary Paget disease of the anus takes its origin from the epidermis or squamous epithelium and may not always evolve into an invasive lesion. In contrast, secondary Paget disease is often linked to an underlying visceral malignancy (eg, colorectal or ovarian carcinoma) and can either present synchronously or metachronously to the primary. Based on limited data, the incidence of synchronous visceral malignancy could be greater than 50% and should be excluded at diagnosis.[21] Occasionally histologically pagetoid extension of cancer cells from an underlying anal or RA is seen in the overlying or immediately adjacent squamous epithelium.

Histologically, Paget disease is classically associated with hyperplastic changes in the involved squamous mucosal surface. Knowledge of such changes assists in making the diagnosis of Paget disease especially during frozen section procedures, to avoid the misdiagnosis of simple squamous dysplasia. There have been efforts to distinguish primary from secondary disease based on immunohistochemical phenotyping; however, data are limited to small case series.[26] It seems that CK7 is a marker of Paget cells, irrespective of their site or an associated visceral malignancy. If it is associated with RA then cells are uniformly immunoreactive to CK20. CK20 expression is seen also in vulvar Paget disease. In those cases, GCDFP15 expression may be helpful; if positive it can lend support toward a nonrectal origin.

The management of Paget disease is usually surgical. The extent of treatment of noninvasive lesions is determined by preoperative mapping of the lesion and intraoperative confirmation by frozen sections to ascertain clear surgical margins. The prognosis of noninvasive Paget disease is good; however, local recurrence is often seen because of the presence of multifocal disease.

Locally invasive perianal Paget disease usually requires a radical surgical approach, although definitive chemoradiotherapy has also been used.[21] Management of secondary Paget disease is directed toward the treatment of the underlying malignancy and these patients have a guarded prognosis.[27,28]

ANORECTAL MELANOMA

Anorectal mucosal melanoma accounts for approximately 0.05% of all colorectal malignancies and 1% of all anal canal cancers.[29,30] It originates in the rectum in 42% and anal canal in 33%, respectively, whereas the primary site cannot be determined in about 25%. Risk factors are not clearly defined apart from the association with human immunodeficiency virus infection.[31–33] Unlike other mucosal melanomas, anorectal site is more common in whites and females with median age of diagnosis at 60 years. Patients typically present with bleeding or a mass, anorectal pain, or change in bowel habit.[34] Occasionally, melanoma is an incidental pathologic finding after hemorrhoidectomy or anal polyp resection. Anorectal mucosal melanoma is pigmented in approximately one-third of cases and at presentation most lesions are greater than 2 mm thick. Regional lymph node involvement is seen in 60% of cases and distant metastases are present at diagnoses in about 30%.[35–38]

Pathology and Staging

Overall 20% of mucosal melanomas are multifocal, compared with less than 5% of cutaneous melanomas and 40% are amelanotic.[39,40] Histologic features are similar to cutaneous melanomas showing a junctional component adjacent to the invasive tumor, which also serves as evidence that the lesion is primary rather than metastatic (**Fig. 4**). The desmoplastic variant may occasionally occur at this site. Diagnosis may be challenging and requires immunohistochemical confirmation with tumor cells expressing S-100, HMB-45, and melan A (see **Fig. 4**). Factors associated with poor prognosis are tumor size and thickness, regional lymph node involvement, presence of perineural invasion, and amelanotic subtype.[37,41,42]

Anorectal melanoma is not addressed by the current American Joint Committee on Cancer staging system. Based on retrospective series, it is categorized as localized disease only, regional lymph node involvement, or distant metastases.[43,44] Survival outcomes from the Surveillance, Epidemiology and End Results database review of 183 patients treated for anorectal mucosal melanoma over a historic period (1973–2003) are presented in **Table 1**.[36]

Management

Locoregional disease

The primary aim of surgery is for curative resection (wide excision) to achieve negative margins. If possible a sphincter-sparing excision is performed; occasionally APR is

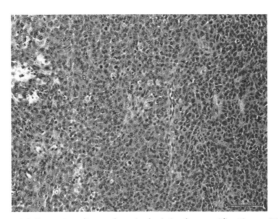

Fig. 4. Melanoma, with hematoxylin and eosin (original magnification ×200) and with S100 immunohistochemical staining. Discohesive sheets of markedly atypical, epithelioid cells with prominent nucleoli and scattered mitoses and apoptotic cells are present in the soft tissue beneath the squamous epithelium. The tumor also showed focal but subtle melanin pigment.

Table 1
Surveillance, Epidemiology and End Results database review for the period 1973–2003 for survival outcomes in patients with anorectal mucosal melanoma

Stage[a]	Median Overall Survival, mo	Survival Rate, %
I (localized disease)	24	26.7
II (regional lymph node involved)	17	9.8
III (distant metastases)	8	0

[a] Defined as per data collection.

necessary for bulky disease or as salvage for patients with local but not systemic recurrence.[45] The impact of the extent of resection on long-term outcome has been reported in a few retrospective case series only. Although there is some evidence lending support to upfront APR providing improved local control at the expense of higher morbidity and detriment to QoL and functional capacity,[42,43] there is no evidence that more extensive surgery is associated with a better OS.[37,46–48] There is no proven role for sentinel lymph node biopsy or elective bilateral inguinal lymph node dissection in the absence of clinical nodal disease.[46,49,50]

Factors associated with a better outcome are R0 resection and tumor stage, based on the Swedish National Cancer Registry dataset. In a published series of 251 patients, the 5-year survival rates following an R0 resection were 19% compared with 6% where local excision was incomplete.[46,47]

Adjuvant therapy

Adjuvant treatment to improve locoregional relapse rate or OS has not been prospectively studied; however, adjuvant radiotherapy is often added to improve local control. The MD Anderson Cancer Center has reported on a series of 54 patients treated during 1989 to 2008 with hypofractionated radiotherapy (25–30 Gy in 5–6 fractions over a 2- to 3-week period) following sphincter-sparing local excision. The radiation was added as an alternative to APR. This approach was associated with local control in 82% of patients with sphincter preservation in 92% but there was no demonstrable impact on OS, with only 30% alive at 5 years.[51] The development of IMRT and VMAT techniques significantly reduces toxicity, which may increase its utility.

Systemic adjuvant therapy is not established in patients with mucosal melanoma. The only randomized evidence comes from a phase II study from China that enrolled 189 patients with resected mucosal melanoma. A total of 56 patients had anorectal melanoma and patients were randomized to observation (n = 21), 1 year of interferon alfa-2b (n = 17), or chemotherapy (n = 18; temozolomide plus cisplatin).[52] The median DFS was significantly prolonged in the chemotherapy arm compared with interferon and observation (20.8 vs 9.4 vs 5.4 months, respectively) as was median OS (49 vs 40 vs 21 months). However, no data have been reported in Western populations.

Metastatic disease

Treatment is based on extrapolation from trials of metastatic cutaneous melanoma. Few patients with melanoma of mucosal origin were enrolled in the clinical trials of modern antimelanoma therapies, with specific exclusion criteria for primaries of mucosal origin.

Approximately 10% of mucosal melanomas harbor the *BRAF* v600E driver mutation and a further 25% have somatic mutations including 9% with *KIT* mutations in exon 11 or 13.[53,54] Among all patients with mucosal melanoma with *BRAF* mutation, anorectal mucosal origin is the most common (20%) primary site.[55,56]

Results from three small phase II trials evaluating the role of imatinib in advanced mucosal melanoma (no breakdown of site of origin stated) harboring somatic alterations of *KIT* demonstrate significant activity[53,57,58] (**Table 2**).

Retrospective analysis from three major US centers demonstrated encouraging activity of the anti-CTLA4 immunotherapy agent ipilimumab in 33 patients with metastatic mucosal melanoma (eight of anorectal origin).[59] Data from 71 patients with metastatic mucosal melanoma (eight of anal origin) from a European extended access program for ipilimumab documented a disease control rate of 36% at median follow-up of 22 months.[60]

A pooled analysis of 121 patients with advanced mucosal melanoma from six trials using the human IgG4 anti-PD-1 monoclonal antibody nivolumab alone or combined with ipilimumab was presented at the 2015 Society of Melanoma Research Conference. A clinically meaningful improvement with monotherapy and combination was demonstrated in the whole group (primary site unstated) with overall response rate for dual therapy of 37%.[61]

PRIMARY LYMPHOMA OF THE ANORECTAL REGION

Anorectal lymphomas are rare comprising only 0.2% of anorectal tumors. Most are non-Hodgkin lymphoma; lymphoma at this site represents 9% of all non-Hodgkin lymphoma.[62,63] Cases of anorectal Hodgkin disease are extremely rare.[64] Anorectal lymphoma is reported to mainly affect young males but this is biased by data relating to the common association with AIDS (mean age, 34 vs 65 in HIV-negative group), particularly when the CD4 count is less than 100 per mm^3. The usage of highly active anti-retroviral therapy has impacted significantly on the incidence of AIDS-associated lymphoma.[65] AIDS-related lymphoma usually presents as extranodal disease and in one-quarter of patients the anorectal region is involved. Patients usually present with a mass or chronic ulceration with or without local lymphadenopathy; however, many patients are normal at examination and have normal initial investigations. In most AIDS-related cases the pathology demonstrates a high-grade large cell immuno-blastic or pleomorphic B-cell lymphoma.[66,67] In patients without HIV, anal lymphoma is more commonly found at older age, is more prevalent in men, and is associated with risk factors including ulcerative colitis or other immunodeficiency conditions. Histologically these are most commonly lower grade B cell histology including mucosal-associated lymphatic tissue.[68]

Management

Patients are treated in line with standard lymphoma management protocols and surgery is restricted to biopsy, although some studies have suggested surgery for

Table 2			
Phase II trials evaluating the role of imatinib in advanced mucosal melanoma			
Trial	Carvajal et al,[53] 2011 N = 25	Hodi et al,[57] 2013 N = 25	Guo et al,[58] 2011 N = 43
Overall response rate	16%	29%[a]	—
Median progression-free survival	12 wk	—	3.5 mo
Median overall survival	46.3 wk	77%	53.5%
Disease control rates	—	—	—

[a] Best objective response rate.

resectable lesions.[63,69,70] Treatment of localized anal lymphoma may involve external beam radiotherapy in addition to chemotherapy. In comparison with the pre–highly active antiretroviral therapy era where OS was 8 months in AIDS-related Diffuse Large Bcell Lymphoma, the current 5-year OS approximates 60% to 80%.[71]

ANAL NEUROENDOCRINE TUMORS

Neuroendocrine cancer can arise anywhere in the body, but neuroendocrine neoplasms of the anorectal region are extremely rare and probably arise from the neuroendocrine cells in colorectal type mucosa, although neuroendocrine cells can be present in anal transitional zone mucosa. Incidental discovery at colonoscopy is increasingly common, as is the case with rectal NETs.[72] A recent analysis of NETs incidence in Ontario, Canada (population 13.6 million) between Jan 1994 and March 2012 documented less than 15 cases of anal origin of a total of 5619 NETs; in comparison there were 690 cases of rectal origin (12.3%) (S. Singh, personal communication, 2016, with permission and disclosure: parts of this material are based on data and information provided by Cancer Care Ontario. The opinions, results, view, and conclusions reported in this paper are those of the authors and do not necessarily reflect those of Cancer Care Ontario. No endorsement by Cancer Care Ontario is intended or should be inferred).[73]

The classification of gastroenteropancreatic neuroendocrine neoplasms has evolved and the World Health Organization endorses the European Neuroendocrine Tumor Society's grading system for neuroendocrine neoplasms of any site within the digestive tract. This is based on the proliferative rate to stratify grade and requires a mitotic count and the Ki-67 labeling index. This system classifies well-differentiated tumors into low-grade (G1) and intermediate-grade (G2) categories; and all poorly differentiated NETs are classified as high-grade (G3) neuroendocrine carcinomas.[74,75] Low-to-intermediate grade NETs can be indolent in their clinical course; however, large tumor size, invasion depth, lymphovascular invasion, and an elevated mitotic rate are associated with poor prognosis.[74,75] Anal NETs seem to behave more aggressively and the rare anal NET portends a poor prognosis.[76–78]

Pathology

Morphologically, well-differentiated NETs display an organoid arrangement of the tumor cells with nesting, trabecular, or gyriform patterns. The cells have round-to-oval nuclei with coarsely stippled chromatin and granular cytoplasm. They display strong and diffuse immunohistochemical reactivity to neuroendocrine markers, such as chromogranin and synaptophysin. Poorly differentiated high-grade neuroendocrine carcinomas have a more sheet-like or diffuse architecture, irregular nuclei, and less cytoplasmic granularity, with patchy or even negligent expression of neuroendocrine markers.[79] Immunohistochemical stains are particularly helpful on biopsy samples when differentiating between usual adenocarcinoma; however, high-grade neuroendocrine carcinomas may be confused with poorly differentiated adenocarcinoma, SCC, or melanoma. Small cell carcinomas of the anal canal may show immune-reactivity for thyroid transcription factor–1 and CK and usually lack staining with synaptophysin and chromogranin and markers of squamous differentiation (34bE12 and p63/4A4). Occasionally a mixed differentiation is present with small cell carcinoma containing dispersed foci of cells with squamous differentiation, usually consisting of less than 5% of the entire tumor specimen, or a mixed differentiation with the presence of adenocarcinoma and neuroendocrine carcinoma cells.[80]

Management

Treatment of anorectal NET is usually determined by size of primary lesion, with surgical excision as the only definitive cure. Tumors that are low grade and are of small size (<1 cm) and depth (confined to the mucosa or submucosa, T1) carry a low risk of metastases and are managed with skilled endoscopic resection. This is preferred for superficial or polypoid lesions; however, there is a risk of positive resection margin.[81] Surgery is usually reserved for lesions 1 to 2 cm with features of invasion or where endoscopic resection is technically difficult. Larger tumors have higher metastatic potential and should undergo complete resection including regional lymph nodes, which could be either APR or anterior resection.[82] 68Ga-DOTATATE PET/computed tomography is used in staging and has high accuracy in detecting bone and soft tissue metastatic disease.[83] Transanal endoscopic microsurgery is an emerging modality where accurate local full-thickness excision of lesions is performed with minimal morbidity.[84] Transanal endoscopic microsurgery in a series of 24 patients resulted in negative resection margins with no local recurrences for patients with either primary lesions or residual disease after endoscopic resection.[85] In selective advanced cases palliative resection can also be considered particularly to debulk the tumor to alleviate symptoms and improve QoL.

Treatment recommendations for management of advanced disease are based on extrapolation from trials of mid-gut NETs because there is a paucity of published data for patients with metastatic colorectal NETs.[86] Somatostatin analogues, peptide-receptor targeted therapy, liver-directed therapies (eg, hepatic bland embolization), radiofrequency ablation and selective internal radiotherapy, interferon alpha, and cytotoxic chemotherapy are used and angiogenesis inhibitors and mTOR inhibitors have recently been added to the therapeutic armamentarium.[82] Treatment in the metastatic setting is usually dictated by the bulk of disease, symptoms, and patient's overall performance status. Aggressive treatment should be considered given the ultimately poor prognosis.

MESENCHYMAL NEOPLASMS

The most common mesenchymal tumors arising in the anal canal are smooth muscle tumors and GIST. Schwannomas, sarcomas related to endometriosis or the mullerian system, and lymphagiomas have also been reported.[6,87,88]

Gastrointestinal Stromal Tumors

Approximately 2% to 8% of anorectal GISTs arise in the anal canal and account for 5% to 10% of all GISTs.[88,89] Morphologically GISTs are spindle cell (65%), epithelioid, or mixed types. A total of 84% of c-kit-positive GISTs stain positively for CD34, with 29% positive for SMA and 4% for S100 protein.[88] In a series of 133 anorectal GISTs including three cases of anal origin, the tumors were histologically similar to gastric and small intestinal GIST with CD117 positive in 96%. Exons 9, 11, and 13 of the c-kit gene were amplified in 29 cases and exon 11 mutations were seen in 17 tumors.[88] DOG-1 is another useful immunohistochemical stain expressed in most GISTs; however, in a report of 12 cases, the single anorectal GIST was not positive.[90–92]

There are no data specifically for anal GIST to suggest a difference from the significant prognostic factors of all GISTs being tumor size and mitotic index. GISTs greater than 5 cm or with greater than 5 mitoses/50 HPFs behave aggressively, whereas size 2 to 5 cm with mitotic count less than 5/HPF have an intermediate risk profile.[68,93]

Surgical resection is the definitive curative treatment. Sphincter preservation must be weighed against recurrence risk because anorectal GISTs could have a variable anatomic relapse pattern. Size and location dictate the extent of resection, with small lesions amenable to mucosal resection; APR is required for more advanced disease.[93–95] MRI is particularly useful for local tumor assessment (**Figs. 5** and **6**). Multiple large studies with long-term follow-up have established the role of adjuvant imatinib therapy in patients with resected GIST, although there is differential efficacy according to subtype of mutation present; no specific profiling of anal GIST mutations have been reported. Data for the anal subset from prospective trials are scant because two of the largest trials of adjuvant imatinib for completely resected GIST by the American College of Surgeons Oncology Group (ACOSOG Z9000 and Z9001) enrolled only 35 anorectal GIST of a total of 751 patients.

BASAL CELL CARCINOMA

BCC of the anus is extremely rare, comprising approximately 0.2% of all anorectal malignancies.[96] Lesions arise at the anal margin and are usually 1 to 2 cm in diameter. BCCs are commonly ulcerated with a raised margin and are often misdiagnosed as anal fissures or hemorrhoids. Histopathologic confirmation is required to distinguish from the basaloid SCC, because this has management implications.[97,98] Wide local excision is the treatment of choice and is curative in most cases; however, APR may be required where the lesion is invading the anal canal and into deeper surrounding tissue. BCCs seldom metastasize and in the two largest series published (Paterson and colleagues,[99] n = 21; Gibson and Ahmed,[100] n = 51), the recurrence rate post wide local excision ranges from 0% to 29% of patients but the cancer-specific survival at 5-year was 100%.

METASTASES TO ANAL CANAL

The anal canal could be a rare site for metastases for any kind of malignancy. In the literature only a few cases have been reported of metastases from breast, lung, colon,

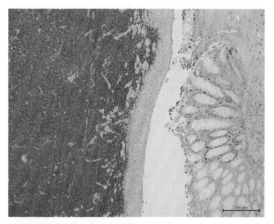

Fig. 5. The malignant cells show strong diffuse staining for S100 (original magnification ×40). Positivity was also demonstrated using a cocktail of antibodies that included HMB-45, Melan-A, and tyrosinase.

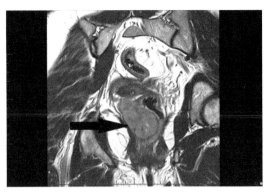

Fig. 6. MRI coronal T2-weighted: primary anorectal GIST (*arrow*).

and pancreatic cancer (**Table 3**).[101–107] Thorough histologic and immunohistochemical analysis is warranted where there is a suspicion of metastases.

SUMMARY

Uncommon neoplasms of the anal canal are associated with significant diagnostic dilemma in clinical practice and a high index of suspicion and particularly pathologic expertise is needed. **Table 4** illustrates some essential morphologic and immunohistochemical properties of uncommon anal canal neoplasms that could be used as a guide. The incidence as with all anal cancers is likely to increase over time, particularly of small, incidental lesions found because of use of more frequent colonoscopy and high-definition MRI. Generally treatment follows that of the same histologic subtype in other anatomic locations rather than usual anal SCC. Surgical intervention is considered as the cornerstone for cure in early and localized disease; however, removal of the anal canal is associated with significant morbidities and QoL issues. Clinical trials in rare anal cancer subtypes are unlikely to be performed but a strong case is made for a centralized global registry/database that could be established under the auspices of the International Rare Care Initiative collaboration.

Table 3			
Published case reports of metastasis to anal canal			
Author/Year	**Demographic Information**	**Site of Primary**	**Histologic and Immunohistochemistry Features**
Takahashi et al,[107] 2011	Case series of 6	Colorectal	Not available
Bochicchio et al,[102] 2012	72 F	Breast	Adenocarcinoma of mammary origin, ER/PR/Her2-ve
Puglisi et al,[103] 2009	88 F	Breast	Invasive lobular carcinoma
Haberstich et al,[104] 2005	78 F	Breast	Ductal carcinoma
Dawson et al,[105] 1985	70 F	Breast	Invasive lobular carcinoma
Kawahara et al,[106] 1994	75 M	Lung	Squamous cell carcinoma
Ejtehadi et al,[101] 2014	79 F	Ampullary	Adenocarcinoma, pancreatobilliary type. CK7/CK17/MUC1 +, (−ve K20/CDX2/MUC2)

Table 4
Histologic identification of rare anal cancer subtypes using morphologic features and immunophenotypic profiles

Tumor	Morphology	Immunohistochemistry Reactivity						
		Keratin	P63	Ki-67	Neuroendocrine Markers[a]	Melanoma Markers[b]	Lymphoma Markers[c]	Other
Adenocarcinoma	Gland forming, mucin producing	−/+	−	−	−	−	−	...
NET								
Carcinoid	Trabecular/organoid No or low proliferative index	−	−	<10%	++	−	−	...
Small cell	Can have squamous differentiation	− (squamous foci+)	− (squamous foci+)	>50%	+/−	−	−	...
High-grade neuroendocrine carcinoma	Can mimic carcinoid but high mitoses ± necrosis	−	−	>30%–50%	+/−	−	−	...
Melanoma	Lesions resemble cutaneous melanoma, pigmentation +/−	−	−	−	−	++	−	...
Non-Hodgkin lymphoma	Large cell immunoblastic or pleomorphic	−	−	−	−	−	++	...
GIST	Cellular tumor with solid growth pattern	−	−	−	−	−	−	CD117 +/− DOG1 CD34, SMA
Sarcoma	Variable depending on type	+/−	−	Variable	−	...	−	Variable

a Synaptophysin, chromogranin.
b Melan, S100, HMB 45.
c CD45, LCA.

REFERENCES

1. Glynne-Jones R, Nilsson PJ, Aschele C, et al. Anal cancer: ESMO-ESSO-ESTRO clinical practice guidelines for diagnosis, treatment and follow-up. Eur J Surg Oncol 2014;40(10):1165–76.
2. Klas JV, Rothenberger DA, Wong WD, et al. Malignant tumors of the anal canal: the spectrum of disease, treatment, and outcomes. Cancer 1999;85(8): 1686–93.
3. Beal KP, Wong D, Guillem JG, et al. Primary adenocarcinoma of the anus treated with combined modality therapy. Dis Colon Rectum 2003;46(10):1320–4.
4. Franklin RA, Giri S, Valasareddy P, et al. Comparative survival of patients with anal adenocarcinoma, squamous cell carcinoma of the anus, and rectal adeno-carcinoma. Clin Colorectal Cancer 2016;15(1):47–53.
5. Fenger C, Frisch M, Marti MC, et al. Tumours of the anal canal. In: Hamilton SR, Aaltonen LA, editors. Pathology and genetics of tumours of the digestive sys-tem. Lyon (France): IARC Publications, International Agency For Research on Cancer; 2000. p. 145–55.
6. Shia J. An update on tumors of the anal canal. Arch Pathol Lab Med 2010; 134(11):1601–11.
7. Koulos J, Symmans F, Chumas J, et al. Human papillomavirus detection in adenocarcinoma of the anus. Mod Pathol 1991;4(1):58–61.
8. Kounalakis N, Artinyan A, Smith D, et al. Abdominal perineal resection improves survival for nonmetastatic adenocarcinoma of the anal canal. Ann Surg Oncol 2009;16(5):1310–5.
9. Edge SB, Byrd DR, Compton CC, et al, editors. American Joint Committee on Cancer staging manual. New York: Springer; 2010. p. 165.
10. Basik M, Rodriguez-Bigas MA, Penetrante R, et al. Prognosis and recurrence patterns of anal adenocarcinoma. Am J Surg 1995;169(2):233–7.
11. Hagihara P, Vazquez MD, Parker JC Jr, et al. Carcinoma of anal-ductal origin: report of a case. Dis Colon Rectum 1976;19(8):694–701.
12. Wong AY, Rahilly MA, Adams W, et al. Mucinous anal gland carcinoma with peri-anal pagetoid spread. Pathology 1998;30(1):1–3.
13. Sakamoto T, Konishi F, Yoshida T, et al. Adenocarcinoma arising from an anal gland: report of a case. Int J Surg Case Rep 2014;5(5):234–6.
14. Hobbs CM, Lowry MA, Owen D, et al. Anal gland carcinoma. Cancer 2001; 92(8):2045–9.
15. Kuroda N, Tanida N, Ohara M, et al. Anal canal adenocarcinoma with MUC5AC expression suggestive of anal gland origin. Med Mol Morphol 2007;40(1):50–3.
16. Anthony T, Simmang C, Lee EL, et al. Perianal mucinous adenocarcinoma. J Surg Oncol 1997;64(3):218–21.
17. Jones EA, Morson BC. Mucinous adenocarcinoma in anorectal fistulae. Histopa-thology 1984;8(2):279–92.
18. Ky A, Sohn N, Weinstein MA, et al. Carcinoma arising in anorectal fistulas of Crohn's disease. Dis Colon Rectum 1998;41(8):992–6.
19. Yeong ML, Wood KP, Scott B, et al. Synchronous squamous and glandular neoplasia of the anal canal. J Clin Pathol 1992;45(3):261–3.
20. Massit H, Edderai M, Saouab R, et al. Adenocarcinoma arising from chronic perianal Crohn's disease: a case report. Pan Afr Med J 2015;22:140.
21. Billingsley KG, Stern LE, Lowy AM, et al. Uncommon anal neoplasms. Surg On-col Clin N Am 2004;13(2):375–88.

22. Papagikos M, Crane CH, Skibber J, et al. Chemoradiation for adenocarcinoma of the anus. Int J Radiat Oncol Biol Phys 2003;55(3):669–78.
23. Belkacemi Y, Berger C, Poortmans P, et al. Management of primary anal canal adenocarcinoma: a large retrospective study from the Rare Cancer Network. Int J Radiat Oncol Biol Phys 2003;56(5):1274–83.
24. Bertelson N, Blumetti J, Cintron J, et al. Anal adenocarcinoma: outcomes in an uncommon malignancy. Am Surg 2015;81(11):1114–7.
25. Crocker HR. Pemphigus vegetans (neumann). Med Chir Trans 1889;72:233–256.1.
26. Goldblum JR, Hart WR. Perianal Paget's disease: a histologic and immunohistochemical study of 11 cases with and without associated rectal adenocarcinoma. Am J Surg Pathol 1998;22(2):170–9.
27. Chanda JJ. Extramammary Paget's disease: prognosis and relationship to internal malignancy. J Am Acad Dermatol 1985;13(6):1009–14.
28. Mehta NJ, Torno R, Sorra T. Extramammary Paget's disease. South Med J 2000;93(7):713–5.
29. Cagir B, Whiteford MH, Topham A, et al. Changing epidemiology of anorectal melanoma. Dis Colon Rectum 1999;42(9):1203–8.
30. Chen H, Cai Y, Liu Y, et al. Incidence, surgical treatment, and prognosis of anorectal melanoma From 1973 to 2011: a population-based SEER analysis. Medicine (Baltimore) 2016;95(7):e2770.
31. Burgi A, Brodine S, Wegner S, et al. Incidence and risk factors for the occurrence of non-AIDS-defining cancers among human immunodeficiency virus-infected individuals. Cancer 2005;104(7):1505–11.
32. Cote TR, Sobin LH. Primary melanomas of the esophagus and anorectum: epidemiologic comparison with melanoma of the skin. Melanoma Res 2009;19(1):58–60.
33. Tariq MU, Ud Din N, Ud Din NF, et al. Malignant melanoma of anorectal region: a clinicopathologic study of 61 cases. Ann Diagn Pathol 2014;18(5):275–81.
34. Goldman S, Glimelius B, Pahlman L. Anorectal malignant melanoma in Sweden. Report of 49 patients. Dis Colon Rectum 1990;33(10):874–7.
35. Chang AE, Karnell LH, Menck HR. The National Cancer Data Base report on cutaneous and noncutaneous melanoma: a summary of 84,836 cases from the past decade. The American College of Surgeons Commission on Cancer and the American Cancer Society. Cancer 1998;83(8):1664–78.
36. Iddings DM, Fleisig AJ, Chen SL, et al. Practice patterns and outcomes for anorectal melanoma in the USA, reviewing three decades of treatment: is more extensive surgical resection beneficial in all patients? Ann Surg Oncol 2010;17(1):40–4.
37. Pessaux P, Pocard M, Elias D, et al. Surgical management of primary anorectal melanoma. Br J Surg 2004;91(9):1183–7.
38. Weinstock MA. Epidemiology and prognosis of anorectal melanoma. Gastroenterology 1993;104(1):174–8.
39. Carvajal RD, Spencer SA, Lydiatt W. Mucosal melanoma: a clinically and biologically unique disease entity. J Natl Compr Canc Netw 2012;10(3):345–56.
40. Lotem M, Anteby S, Peretz T, et al. Mucosal melanoma of the female genital tract is a multifocal disorder. Gynecol Oncol 2003;88(1):45–50.
41. Cooper PH, Mills SE, Allen MS Jr. Malignant melanoma of the anus: report of 12 patients and analysis of 255 additional cases. Dis Colon Rectum 1982;25(7):693–703.

42. Brady MS, Kavolius JP, Quan SH. Anorectal melanoma. A 64-year experience at Memorial Sloan-Kettering Cancer Center. Dis Colon Rectum 1995;38(2):146–51.
43. Roumen RM. Anorectal melanoma in The Netherlands: a report of 63 patients. Eur J Surg Oncol 1996;22(6):598–601.
44. Australian Cancer Network Melanoma Guidelines Revision Working Party. Clinical Practice Guidelines for the Management of Melanoma in Australia and New Zealand. Cancer Council Australia and Australian Cancer Network, Sydney and New Zealand Guidelines Group, Wellington; 2008. Available at: http://www.cancer.org.au/content/pdf/HealthProfessionals/ClinicalGuidelines/ClinicalPractice Guidelines-ManagementofMelanoma.pdf. Accessed April 5, 2016.
45. Matsuda A, Miyashita M, Matsumoto S, et al. Abdominoperineal resection provides better local control but equivalent overall survival to local excision of anorectal malignant melanoma: a systematic review. Ann Surg 2015;261(4):670–7.
46. Yeh JJ, Shia J, Hwu WJ, et al. The role of abdominoperineal resection as surgical therapy for anorectal melanoma. Ann Surg 2006;244(6):1012–7.
47. Nilsson PJ, Ragnarsson-Olding BK. Importance of clear resection margins in anorectal malignant melanoma. Br J Surg 2010;97(1):98–103.
48. Droesch JT, Flum DR, Mann GN. Wide local excision or abdominoperineal resection as the initial treatment for anorectal melanoma? Am J Surg 2005;189(4):446–9.
49. Tien HY, McMasters KM, Edwards MJ, et al. Sentinel lymph node metastasis in anal melanoma: a case report. Int J Gastrointest Cancer 2002;32(1):53–6.
50. Perez DR, Trakarnsanga A, Shia J, et al. Locoregional lymphadenectomy in the surgical management of anorectal melanoma. Ann Surg Oncol 2013;20(7):2339–44.
51. Kelly P, Zagars GK, Cormier JN, et al. Sphincter-sparing local excision and hypofractionated radiation therapy for anorectal melanoma: a 20-year experience. Cancer 2011;117(20):4747–55.
52. Lian B, Si L, Cui C, et al. Phase II randomized trial comparing high-dose IFN-alpha2b with temozolomide plus cisplatin as systemic adjuvant therapy for resected mucosal melanoma. Clin Cancer Res 2013;19(16):4488–98.
53. Carvajal RD, Antonescu CR, Wolchok JD, et al. KIT as a therapeutic target in metastatic melanoma. JAMA 2011;305(22):2327–34.
54. Curtin JA, Busam K, Pinkel D, et al. Somatic activation of KIT in distinct subtypes of melanoma. J Clin Oncol 2006;24(26):4340–6.
55. Si L, Wang X, Guo J. Genotyping of mucosal melanoma. Chin Clin Oncol 2014;3(3):34.
56. Omholt K, Grafstrom E, Kanter-Lewensohn L, et al. KIT pathway alterations in mucosal melanomas of the vulva and other sites. Clin Cancer Res 2011;17(12):3933–42.
57. Hodi FS, Corless CL, Giobbie-Hurder A, et al. Imatinib for melanomas harboring mutationally activated or amplified KIT arising on mucosal, acral, and chronically sun-damaged skin. J Clin Oncol 2013;31(26):3182–90.
58. Guo J, Si L, Kong Y, et al. Phase II, open-label, single-arm trial of imatinib mesylate in patients with metastatic melanoma harboring c-Kit mutation or amplification. J Clin Oncol 2011;29(21):2904–9.
59. Postow MA, Luke JJ, Bluth MJ, et al. Ipilimumab for patients with advanced mucosal melanoma. Oncologist 2013;18(6):726–32.
60. Del Vecchio M, Di Guardo L, Ascierto PA, et al. Efficacy and safety of ipilimumab 3mg/kg in patients with pretreated, metastatic, mucosal melanoma. Eur J Cancer 2014;50(1):121–7.

61. Larkin J, D'Angelo S, Sosman JA, et al. Efficacy and safety of nivolumab (NIVO) monotherapy in the treatment of advanced mucosal melanoma (MEL). Pigment Cell Melanoma Res 2015;28(6):789.
62. Shepherd NA, Hall PA, Coates PJ, et al. Primary malignant lymphoma of the colon and rectum. A histopathological and immunohistochemical analysis of 45 cases with clinicopathological correlations. Histopathology 1988;12(3):235–52.
63. Cuffy M, Abir F, Longo WE. Management of less common tumors of the colon, rectum, and anus. Clin Colorectal Cancer 2006;5(5):327–37.
64. Ambrosio MR, Rocca BJ, Barone A, et al. Primary anorectal Hodgkin lymphoma: report of a case and review of the literature. Hum Pathol 2014;45(3):648–52.
65. Diamond C, Taylor TH, Aboumrad T, et al. Changes in acquired immunodeficiency syndrome-related non-Hodgkin lymphoma in the era of highly active antiretroviral therapy: incidence, presentation, treatment, and survival. Cancer 2006;106(1):128–35.
66. Heise W, Arasteh K, Mostertz P, et al. Malignant gastrointestinal lymphomas in patients with AIDS. Digestion 1997;58(3):218–24.
67. Ioachim HL, Antonescu C, Giancotti F, et al. EBV-associated anorectal lymphomas in patients with acquired immune deficiency syndrome. Am J Surg Pathol 1997;21(9):997–1006.
68. Peralta EA. Rare anorectal neoplasms: gastrointestinal stromal tumor, carcinoid, and lymphoma. Clin Colon Rectal Surg 2009;22(2):107–14.
69. Zighelboim J, Larson MV. Primary colonic lymphoma. Clinical presentation, histopathologic features, and outcome with combination chemotherapy. J Clin Gastroenterol 1994;18(4):291–7.
70. Fan CW, Changchien CR, Wang JY, et al. Primary colorectal lymphoma. Dis Colon Rectum 2000;43(9):1277–82.
71. Rubinstein PG, Aboulafia DM, Zloza A. Malignancies in HIV/AIDS: from epidemiology to therapeutic challenges. AIDS 2014;28(4):453–65.
72. Gastrointestinal Pathology Study Group of Korean Society of Pathologists, Cho MY, Kim JM, Sohn JH, et al. Current trends of the incidence and pathological diagnosis of gastroenteropancreatic neuroendocrine tumors (GEP-NETs) in Korea 2000-2009: multicenter study. Cancer Res Treat 2012;44(3):157–65.
73. Hallet J, Law CH, Cukier M, et al. Exploring the rising incidence of neuroendocrine tumors: a population-based analysis of epidemiology, metastatic presentation, and outcomes. Cancer 2015;121(4):589–97.
74. Klimstra DS, Modlin IR, Coppola D, et al. The pathologic classification of neuroendocrine tumors: a review of nomenclature, grading, and staging systems. Pancreas 2010;39(6):707–12.
75. Rindi G, Arnold R, Bosman FT, et al. Nomenclature and classification of neuroendocrine neoplasms of the digestive system. In: Bosman TF, Carneiro F, Hruban RH, et al, editors. WHO classification of tumours of the digestive system. 4th edition. Lyon (France): International Agency for Research on Cancer (IARC); 2010. p. 13.
76. Sorbye H, Strosberg J, Baudin E, et al. Gastroenteropancreatic high-grade neuroendocrine carcinoma. Cancer 2014;120(18):2814–23.
77. Simon SR, Fox K. Neuroendocrine carcinoma of the colon. Correct diagnosis is important. J Clin Gastroenterol 1993;17(4):304–7.
78. Modlin IM, Lye KD, Kidd M. A 5-decade analysis of 13,715 carcinoid tumors. Cancer 2003;97(4):934–59.

79. Washington MK, Tang LH, Berlin J, et al. Protocol for the examination of specimens from patients with neuroendocrine tumors (carcinoid tumors) of the stomach. Arch Pathol Lab Med 2010;134(2):187–91.
80. Tang LH, Untch BR, Reidy DL, et al. Well-differentiated neuroendocrine tumors with a morphologically apparent high-grade component: a pathway distinct from poorly differentiated neuroendocrine carcinomas. Clin Cancer Res 2016;22(4): 1011–7.
81. Kobayashi K, Katsumata T, Yoshizawa S, et al. Indications of endoscopic polypectomy for rectal carcinoid tumors and clinical usefulness of endoscopic ultrasonography. Dis Colon Rectum 2005;48(2):285–91.
82. Caplin M, Sundin A, Nillson O, et al. ENETS Consensus Guidelines for the management of patients with digestive neuroendocrine neoplasms: colorectal neuroendocrine neoplasms. Neuroendocrinology 2012;95(2):88–97.
83. Skoura E, Michopoulou S, Mohmaduvesh M, et al. The impact of 68Ga-DOTATATE PET/CT imaging on management of patients with neuroendocrine tumors: experience from a National Referral Center in the United Kingdom. J Nucl Med 2016;57(1):34–40.
84. Middleton PF, Sutherland LM, Maddern GJ. Transanal endoscopic microsurgery: a systematic review. Dis Colon Rectum 2005;48(2):270–84.
85. Kumar AS, Sidani SM, Kolli K, et al. Transanal endoscopic microsurgery for rectal carcinoids: the largest reported United States experience. Colorectal Dis 2012;14(5):562–6.
86. Anthony LB, Strosberg JR, Klimstra DS, et al. The NANETS consensus guidelines for the diagnosis and management of gastrointestinal neuroendocrine tumors (nets): well-differentiated nets of the distal colon and rectum. Pancreas 2010;39(6):767–74.
87. Val-Bernal JF, Mayorga M, Diego C, et al. Pedunculated polypoid lymphangioma of the anal canal. Pathol Int 2008;58(7):442–4.
88. Miettinen M, Furlong M, Sarlomo-Rikala M, et al. Gastrointestinal stromal tumors, intramural leiomyomas, and leiomyosarcomas in the rectum and anus: a clinicopathologic, immunohistochemical, and molecular genetic study of 144 cases. Am J Surg Pathol 2001;25(9):1121–33.
89. DeMatteo RP, Lewis JJ, Leung D, et al. Two hundred gastrointestinal stromal tumors: recurrence patterns and prognostic factors for survival. Ann Surg 2000; 231(1):51–8.
90. Novelli M, Rossi S, Rodriguez-Justo M, et al. DOG1 and CD117 are the antibodies of choice in the diagnosis of gastrointestinal stromal tumours. Histopathology 2010;57(2):259–70.
91. Miettinen M, Wang ZF, Lasota J. DOG1 antibody in the differential diagnosis of gastrointestinal stromal tumors: a study of 1840 cases. Am J Surg Pathol 2009; 33(9):1401–8.
92. Solomon R, van Wijk R, Rossouw N. DOG-1: a breed showing K9 excellence. Available at: http://www.leicabiosystems.com/pathologyleaders/dog-1-a-breed-showing-k9-excellence/. Accessed April 5, 2016.
93. Hassan I, You YN, Shyyan R, et al. Surgically managed gastrointestinal stromal tumors: a comparative and prognostic analysis. Ann Surg Oncol 2008;15(1):52–9.
94. Walsh TH, Mann CV. Smooth muscle neoplasms of the rectum and anal canal. Br J Surg 1984;71(8):597–9.
95. Changchien CR, Wu MC, Tasi WS, et al. Evaluation of prognosis for malignant rectal gastrointestinal stromal tumor by clinical parameters and immunohistochemical staining. Dis Colon Rectum 2004;47(11):1922–9.

96. Nielsen OV, Jensen SL. Basal cell carcinoma of the anus-a clinical study of 34 cases. Br J Surg 1981;68(12):856–7.
97. Patil DT, Goldblum JR, Billings SD. Clinicopathological analysis of basal cell carcinoma of the anal region and its distinction from basaloid squamous cell carcinoma. Mod Pathol 2013;26(10):1382–9.
98. Moore HG, Guillem JG. Anal neoplasms. Surg Clin North Am 2002;82(6): 1233–51.
99. Paterson CA, Young-Fadok TM, Dozois RR. Basal cell carcinoma of the perianal region: 20-year experience. Dis Colon Rectum 1999;42(9):1200–2.
100. Gibson GE, Ahmed I. Perianal and genital basal cell carcinoma: a clinicopathologic review of 51 cases. J Am Acad Dermatol 2001;45(1):68–71.
101. Ejtehadi F, Chatzizacharias NA, Brais RJ, et al. Colonic and anal metastases from pancreato-biliary malignancies. World J Gastroenterol 2014;20(13): 3693–7.
102. Bochicchio A, Tartarone A, Ignomirelli O, et al. Anal metastasis from breast cancer: a case report and review of the literature. Future Oncol 2012;8(3):333–6.
103. Puglisi M, Varaldo E, Assalino M, et al. Anal metastasis from recurrent breast lobular carcinoma: a case report. World J Gastroenterol 2009;15(11):1388–90.
104. Haberstich R, Tuech JJ, Wilt M, et al. Anal localization as first manifestation of metastatic ductal breast carcinoma. Tech Coloproctol 2005;9(3):237–8.
105. Dawson PM, Hershman MJ, Wood CB. Metastatic carcinoma of the breast in the anal canal. Postgrad Med J 1985;61(722):1081.
106. Kawahara K, Akamine S, Takahashi T, et al. Anal metastasis from carcinoma of the lung: report of a case. Surg Today 1994;24(12):1101–3.
107. Takahashi H, Ikeda M, Takemasa I, et al. Anal metastasis of colorectal carcinoma origin: implications for diagnosis and treatment strategy. Dis Colon Rectum 2011;54(4):472–81.

Printed and bound by CPI Group (UK) Ltd, Croydon, CR0 4YY

03/10/2024

01040398-0019